Sparkson's

ILLUSTRATED

ECG

INTERPRETATION

— 2ND EDITION —

Written and illustrated
by Jorge Muniz, PA-C

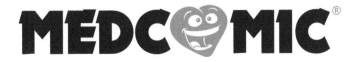

ISBN: 978-0-9966513-7-0

Published by Medcomic, LLC.

Director, designer, manager, editor, illustrator, author: Jorge Muniz

Connect and share:

www.facebook.com/MedcomicWorld

www.twitter.com/Medcomic

www.instagram.com/Medcomic

www.Sparkson.com

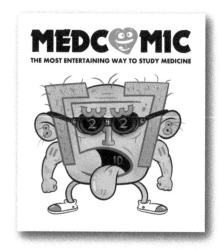

Also from Jorge Muniz:

Medcomic: The Most Entertaining Way to Study Medicine

www.Medcomic.com

This book is dedicated with love to my Mom and Dad,

Carmen Jannette Muniz and Jorge Alberto Muniz.

- Jorge Alexis Muniz

PREFACE

Electrocardiography is an inherently visual subject. Lines are plotted on standardized boxes and measured for deviations from the norm. Even a brief scan over an ECG can provide potentially life-saving information. However, there's more to ECG interpretation than meets the eye. An epic adventure is hidden within these graphs. The pages that follow reveal the full story with vivid illustrations and a memorable cast of characters. You'll learn the essentials of ECG interpretation along the way.

Writing and illustrating my first book, *Medcomic: The Most Entertaining Way to Study Medicine*, has given me unique insight on how to create images that "stick" in the brain of a student. A delicate balance of creativity, consideration, and expertise is needed to create effective mnemonic devices. Care should be taken to avoid making a mnemonic device that is more of a gimmick than a useful learning tool. *Sparkson's Illustrated Guide to ECG Interpretation* represents an evolution in the techniques I've been developing over the past several years as a clinician, artist, and educator.

The format of this book is unconventional and there's an emphasis on reinforcing the material through the use of humorous imagery. Given the scope of the book, you'll likely discover something new when reexamining the material. The artwork is highly memorable because it carries a spirit of personification, hyperbole, and metaphor not found in standard medical textbooks.

Furthermore, *Sparkson's Illustrated Guide to ECG Interpretation* is unique in that it utilizes a main cartoon character as a teaching tool. We may call this mnemonic device the "Medcomic Protagonist." I propose that a unique lead character, with humorous cartoon qualities, can guide a student to learn a great amount of complex medical information with relative ease. Sparkson is a shining example of our first great Medcomic Protagonist.

Emotion plays a significant role in the cartoons I create and it's a quality showcased by Sparkson and his supporting cast. You'll find that the characters weave a thread of entertainment through the entire text. This thread stitches together the educational aspects of the material to create a cohesive whole. There is an element of surprise to each section of the book, and all of these qualities are designed to exponentially enhance the learning experience.

Although we may not realize it, we absorb information from art quite frequently. You may learn, for example, the lyrics to your favorite song as you enjoy the music. This is an effortless learning process that can be adapted to cartoons for higher education. If the art wins you over, the information it contains should be easy to digest. The analogy can be described with the following equation:

$$\frac{\text{Music}}{\text{Lyrics}} = \frac{\text{Cartoons}}{\text{ECG interpretation}}$$

This textbook has two goals. The first is to create a learning experience that eliminates the burden associated with rote memorization. The book includes the most important topics you need to know for ECG interpretation and will serve as a valuable reference. The second goal is to design a book that can also stand on its own as a work of art and entertainment. I didn't want to make a book about the heart without putting my heart in it too. I hope you find it to be a source of inspiration. Enjoy!

Jorge Muniz, PA-C

CONTENTS

Overture

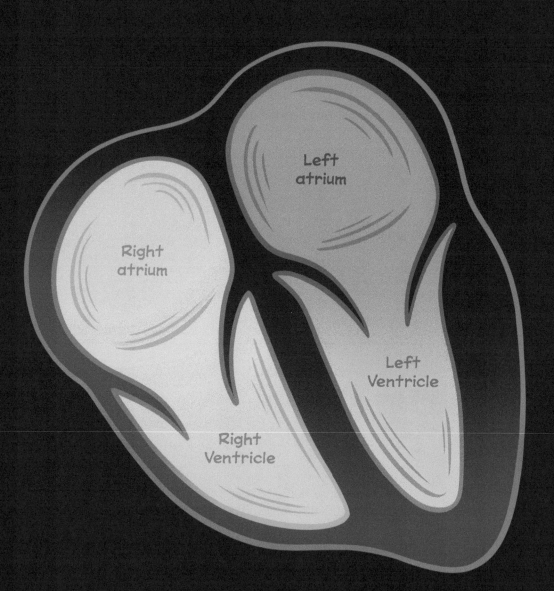

CHAPTER 1

ANATOMY AND PHYSIOLOGY

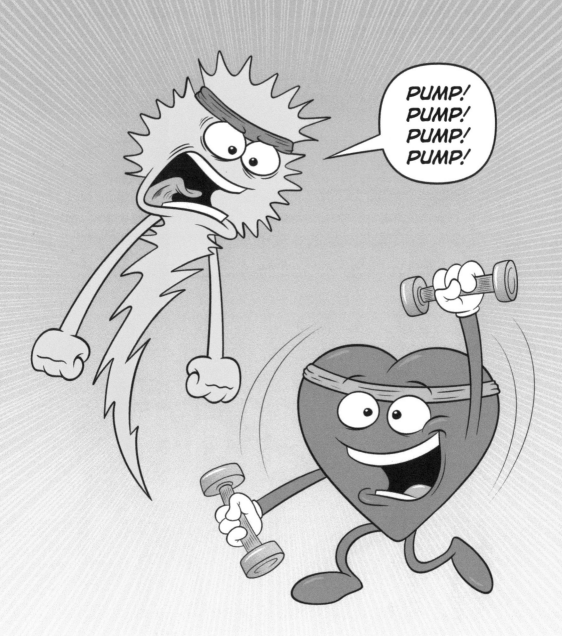

THE heart requires electrical stimulation in order to pump blood throughout the body via the circulatory system. This electrical activity is recorded by the electrocardiogram (ECG), which provides crucial information for establishing many cardiac diagnoses. An ECG machine utilizes skin sensors called electrodes to detect the heart's electrical activity over a short period of time. Details about the heart's structure and function can be inferred from the recording, which is inscribed on a ruled paper strip. This recorded pattern is commonly referred to as an ECG tracing.

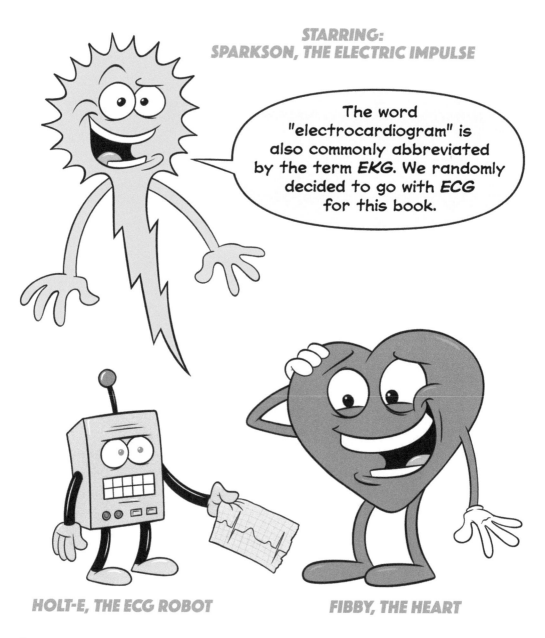

STARRING:
SPARKSON, THE ELECTRIC IMPULSE

The word "electrocardiogram" is also commonly abbreviated by the term *EKG*. We randomly decided to go with *ECG* for this book.

HOLT-E, THE ECG ROBOT

FIBBY, THE HEART

The Heart Cells

Myocardial cells are electrically polarized in their resting state. This means that their interiors are negatively charged with respect to the outside surface.

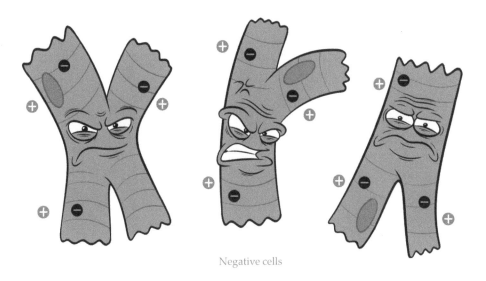

Negative cells

Cardiac cells undergo *depolarization* when ions cross the cell membrane and their interiors become positive, allowing them to contract.

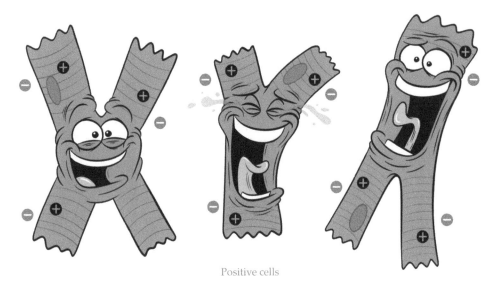

Positive cells

Take a moment to imagine all of the cells in your heart laughing and contracting.

A wave of depolarization is propagated from cell to cell across the entire heart. This wave spreads concentrically, like that of a pebble dropped at the center of a lake. The myocardial cells undergo *repolarization* as the cells return to their (negative) resting state.

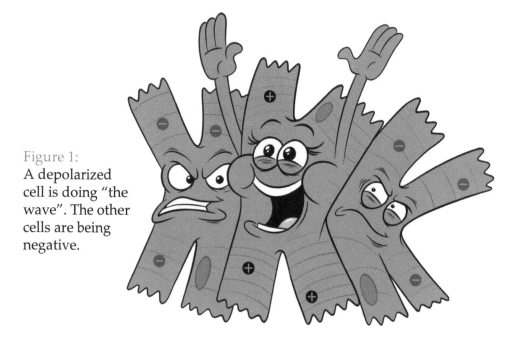

Figure 1:
A depolarized cell is doing "the wave". The other cells are being negative.

The different patterns seen on an ECG are manifestations of the electrical process of depolarization and repolarization in myocardial cells. These processes occur as charged particles called ions pass in and out of the cell.

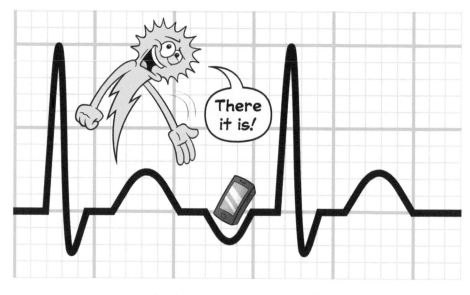

There it is!

Sparkson travels back from page 132

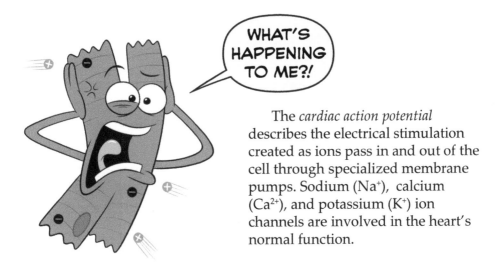

The *cardiac action potential* describes the electrical stimulation created as ions pass in and out of the cell through specialized membrane pumps. Sodium (Na^+), calcium (Ca^{2+}), and potassium (K^+) ion channels are involved in the heart's normal function.

Typical Action Potential of a Contractile Cell

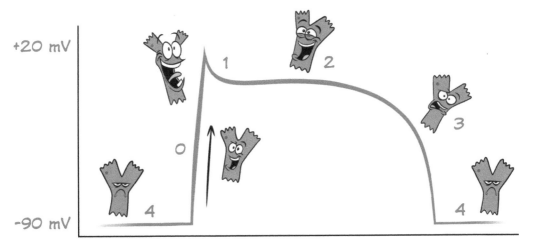

- **Phase 0:** The opening of fast sodium channels is responsible for the rapid depolarization of the cell. The cell quickly becomes positive (and laughs uncontrollably).

- **Phase 1:** Partial repolarization occurs as sodium channels close and potassium flows out of the cell.

- **Phase 2:** A slow influx of calcium causes a plateau phase as potassium continues to leave the cell.

- **Phase 3:** Repolarization occurs as calcium channels close and potassium exits the cell. The cell is becoming negative again.

- **Phase 4:** The cell is at the resting potential.

The Refractory Period

After a cardiac cell has depolarized there is a period of time in which it won't respond to any other stimuli. This is called the refractory period and it correlates with phases 0-3 of the cardiac action potential.

The concept of the refractory period is very important. It helps explain the mechanism behind why many abnormalities manifest on an ECG tracing. Understanding this topic well now will make learning about ECGs much easier in the future.

An *absolute* refractory period, in which absolutely no other stimulus will excite the cell, begins in phase 0 and into part of phase 3. Phase 3 is of particular interest to us, which represents repolarization. This phase includes a *relative* refractory period towards the end in which a strong enough stimulus could potentially excite the cell. A variety of ECG abnormalities correspond with repolarization and the concept of refractoriness.

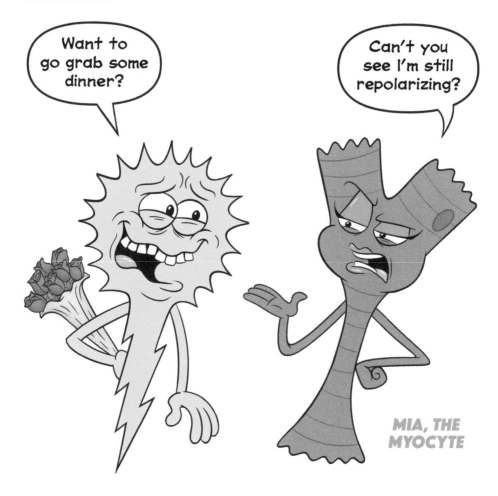

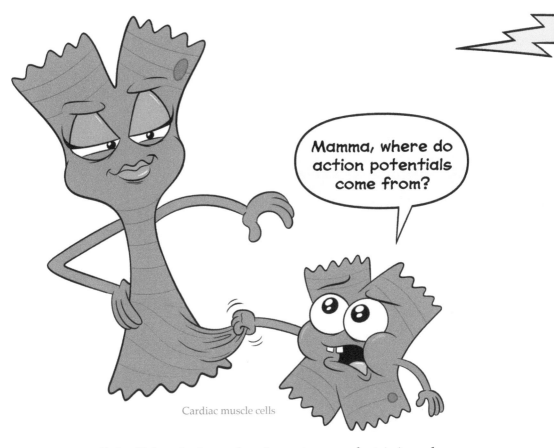

Cardiac muscle cells

A myocardial cell depolarizes when it receives an electric impulse from a neighboring cell, which propagates the action potential. In contrast, a *pacemaker cell* is able to generate an action potential independently from any other cells. This innate ability to spontaneously depolarize is known as *automaticity*. Pacemaker cells thus serve as the electrical power source of the heart. Each spontaneous depolarization initiates the wave of electrical conduction that allows the heart to complete a cycle of contraction and relaxation.

The *sinoatrial (SA) node*, or sinus node, is the primary pacemaker site within the heart and establishes the normal electrical pattern known as sinus rhythm. The SA node is located at the top of the right atrial wall. Other cells in the heart also have the potential to become pacemakers, and these areas of the heart are known as *automaticity foci*.

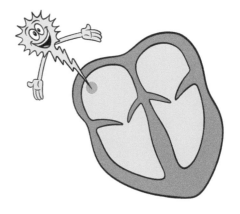

Unlike regular cardiomyocytes, pacemaker cells do not have a stable resting potential (phase 4). Instead, there is a constant fluctuation in polarity as the cell depolarizes and repolarizes at a regular rhythm. Essentially, the action potential of a pacemaker cell differs from that of a cardiomyocyte in that phases 1 and 2 are absent and phase 4 is unstable.

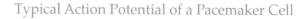

Typical Action Potential of a Pacemaker Cell

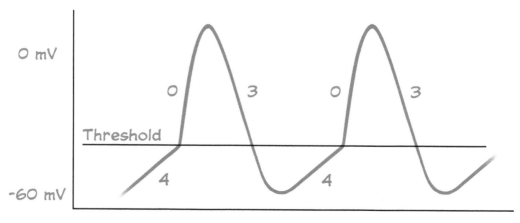

- **Phase 4:** Unique sodium channels called *funny channels* (I_f) open in response to hyperpolarization (a state in which the interior of the cell is very negative), allowing sodium to enter the cell and drive the pacemaker potential up towards the threshold. Potassium channels begin to close, which limits the amount of potassium that can exit the cell. In addition, transient calcium channels open to push the pacemaker potential to the threshold.

- **Phase 0:** A different set of calcium channels open once the threshold is reached, known as long-lasting (L-type) calcium channels. The influx of calcium ions during this phase produces the action potential.

- **Phase 3:** Repolarization occurs as potassium channels open and potassium ions leave the cell. Hyperpolarization stimulates phase 4 to begin again and the cycle repeats.

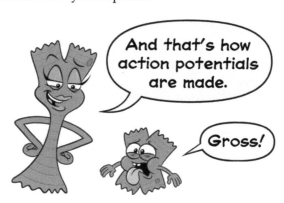

The Atrial Conduction System

The SA node initiates a wave of depolarization that is sent outward in every direction. However, the heart is hard-wired to propagate the bulk of electricity through specific routes.

Electric impulses from the SA node depolarize both atria simultaneously through the atrial conduction system. It consists of three internodal tracts and an additional branch called Bachmann's bundle, which conducts impulses to the left atrium. The three internodal tracts travel from the SA node to the atrioventricular (AV) node and are known as the anterior, middle, and posterior internodal tracts.

These are considered to be the fastest routes for conduction through the atria. However, general excitation does also spread from cell to cell throughout the entire atrial myocardium.

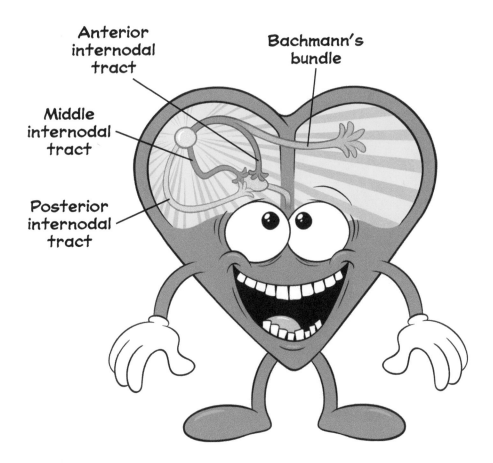

Anterior internodal tract

Bachmann's bundle

Middle internodal tract

Posterior internodal tract

The Cardiac Conduction System

The cardiac conduction system is composed of electrical conducting cells which allow for the rapid transmission of electric impulses throughout the myocardium. These electrical pathways are essential to the organized rhythmic contraction of the heart.

From the SA node, electricity travels through the AV node, bundle of His, right bundle branch, *left bundle branch, and Purkinje fibers.

The Purkinje fibers arise from the right and left bundle branches distally and spread throughout the subendocardium.

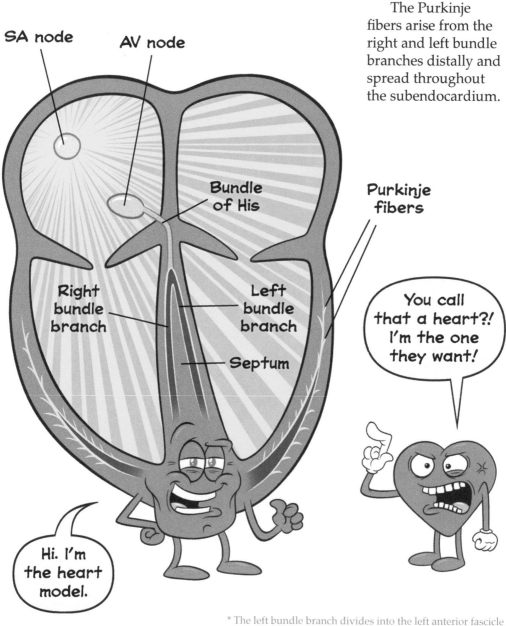

* The left bundle branch divides into the left anterior fascicle and left posterior fascicle (not pictured).

As the left bundle branch travels down the interventricular septum, it divides into the left anterior fascicle and the left posterior fascicle. These fascicles lead to the Purkinje fibers that innervate the left ventricle.

The left anterior fascicle travels anteriorly and superiorly. It is much thinner compared to the left posterior fascicle. The left posterior fascicle is a fan-like structure that travels posteriorly and inferiorly.

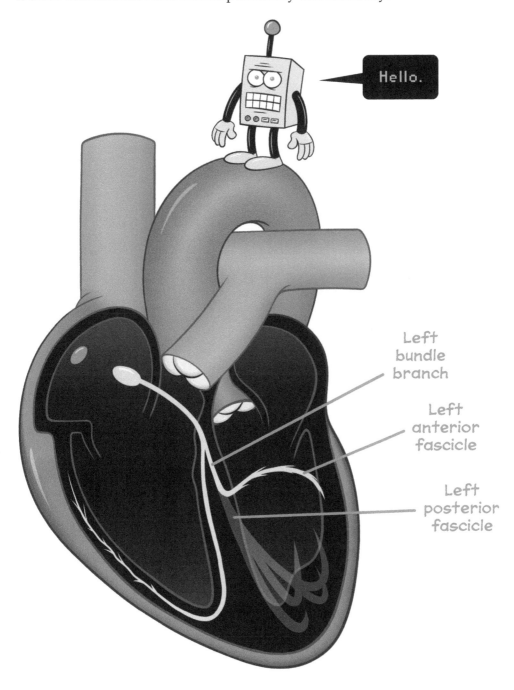

The Heart as a Pump

The cardiovascular system delivers oxygen and nutrients to all of the cells in the body. This is accomplished by the pumping action of the heart, which consists of four main chambers: two atria and two ventricles. The atria contract to empty blood into their corresponding ventricles. The left ventricle pumps blood to the body (systemic circulation), and the right ventricle pumps blood to the lungs (pulmonary circulation). Veins bring oxygen-poor blood towards the heart, while arteries take oxygen-rich blood away from the heart. Blood circulates through this system continuously, receiving oxygen in the lungs and delivering it to the peripheral tissues.

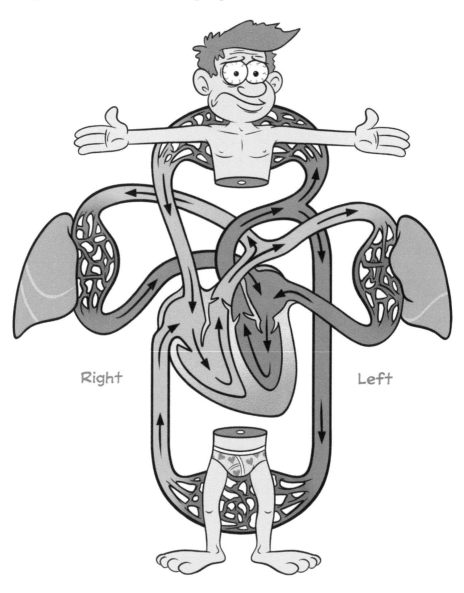

Right   Left

Cardiac Output

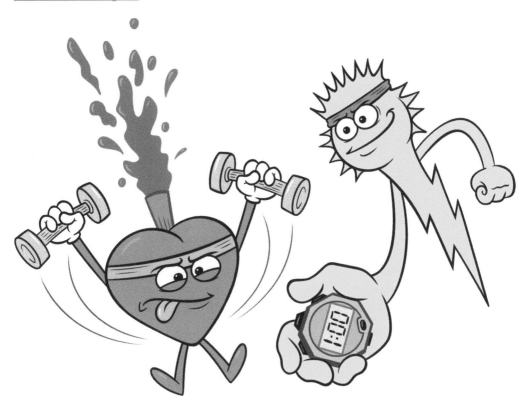

Cardiac output (CO) is the amount of blood pumped by the heart in one minute. It is measured by multiplying the heart rate (HR) by the stroke volume (SV). *Stroke volume* represents the amount of blood ejected by the ventricle with each contraction.

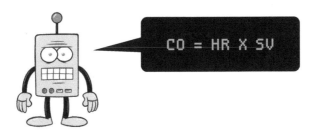

The percentage of blood ejected from the ventricle with each contraction is known as the ejection fraction (EF). A *cardiomyopathy* is a disease of the heart muscle that may cause a low ejection fraction. A worsening cardiomyopathy can lead to heart failure and abnormal heart rhythms.

Heart Valves

Blood flows through a normal pumping heart in one direction. Four valves prevent the backward flow of blood in the heart. These valves open and close depending on pressure changes within the atria and ventricles as the heart contracts.

The two atrioventricular (AV) valves, one located between each atrium and ventricle, prevent the backflow of blood into the atria when the ventricles contract (systole). The tricuspid valve is on the right side and has three flaps. The mitral valve is on the left side and has two flaps.

The AV valves also function to electrically insulate the ventricles from the atria, which allows the AV node to be the dominant pathway in the electrical conduction system when depolarization reaches the interventricular septum.

The two semilunar (SL) valves, consisting of the aortic valve and the pulmonary valve, prevent the backflow of blood into the ventricles. Each valve has three pocket-like cusps which fill with blood and close during ventricular relaxation (diastole).

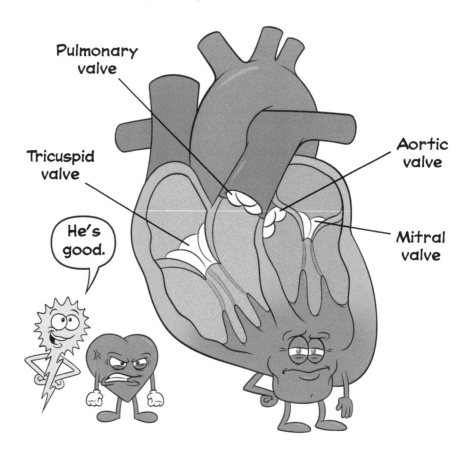

Let's follow Sparkson as he travels through the heart's electrical conduction system during one heartbeat.

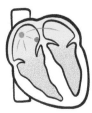

The SA node, located in the upper wall of the right atrium, initiates cardiac conduction by generating an electric impulse that causes both of the atria to contract simultaneously. The normal sinus discharge rate is 60 to 100 times per minute.

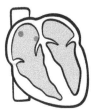

The electric impulse is propagated through the atrial conduction system to the AV node, where there is a brief delay of about 0.12 seconds. This pause allows time for the blood in the atria to enter the ventricles.

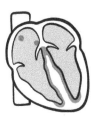

Conduction then sweeps rapidly through the bundle of His and divides into the left and right bundle branches, which are located in the interventricular septum. The wave of depolarization continues towards the apex of the heart.

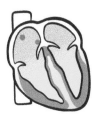

Depolarization sweeps up from the right bundle branch and left anterior and posterior fascicles. The Purkinje fibers conduct the impulse from the apex up through the ventricular myocardium, which causes both ventricles to contract simultaneously.

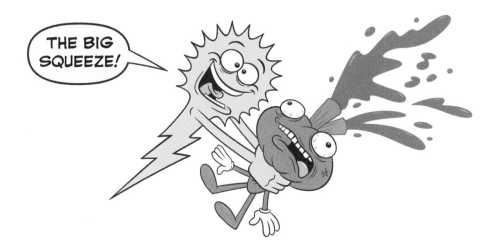

Sparkson's Summary: Chapter 1

- The human heart consists of four main chambers: two atria and two larger ventricles.

- Tricuspid valve: located between the right atrium and right ventricle.

- Mitral valve: located between the left atrium and left ventricle.

- The right ventricle contracts to pump deoxygenated blood through the pulmonary valve to the lungs.

- The left ventricle contracts to push oxygenated blood through the aortic valve and into the body's systemic circulation.

- Cardiac output: the amount of blood pumped by the heart in one minute (CO = HR x SV).

- Ions pass in and out of myocardial cells, causing them to contract and relax. This allows the heart to function as a pump.

- Cardiac action potential: a graphical representation of the change in voltage that occurs as sodium, calcium, and potassium ions cause depolarization and repolarization across cells.

- Refractory period: the period of time after depolarization during which a cardiac cell will not respond to any other stimuli.

- SA node: the heart's primary pacemaker, located at the top of the right atrial wall.

- The main components of the cardiac conduction system include the SA node, AV node, bundle of His, right bundle branch, left bundle branch, left anterior fascicle, left posterior fascicle, and Purkinje fibers.

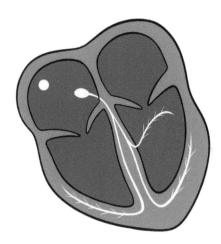

CHAPTER 2

ECG BASICS

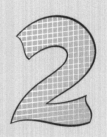

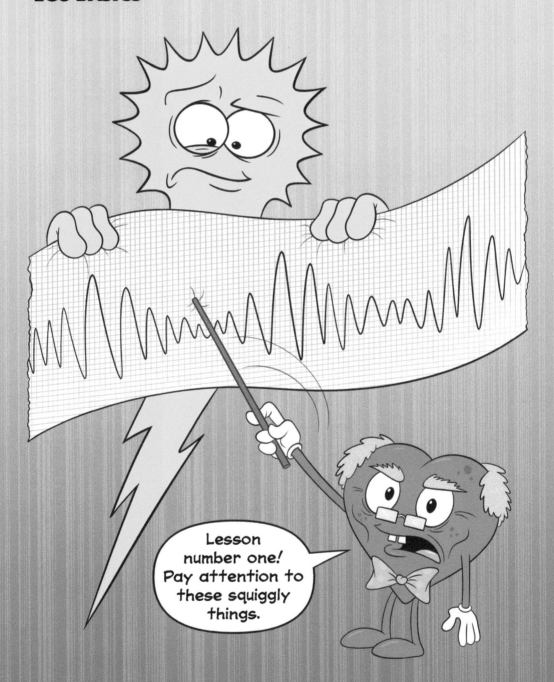

Graphing the ECG

The heart's electrical activity is recorded on special graph paper. This paper is divided into boxes which allow us to make quick measurements of an ECG tracing. Thin lines form small boxes of 1x1 millimeter (mm), and thick lines form larger boxes of 5x5 mm.

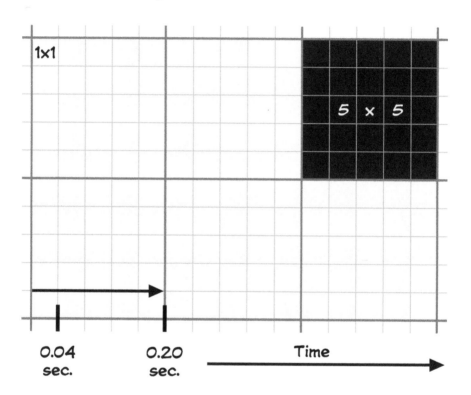

The ECG paper speed is typically standardized to 25 mm per second. Therefore, each 1 mm box represents a span of 0.04 seconds, while each large box that includes five small boxes represents 0.20 seconds.

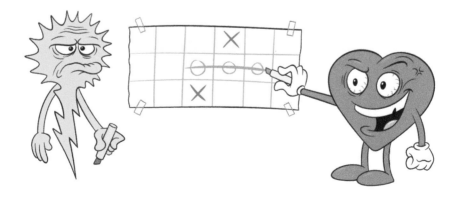

ECG tracings reflect the electrical activity of the heart in the form of *waves*, along with lines connecting the waves known as *segments*. Waves are identified as upward or downward deflections relative to the ECG's baseline (also known as the *isoelectric line*). When a wave is recorded in an upward direction it is known as a *positive* deflection. A *negative* deflection occurs when a wave moves in a downward direction.

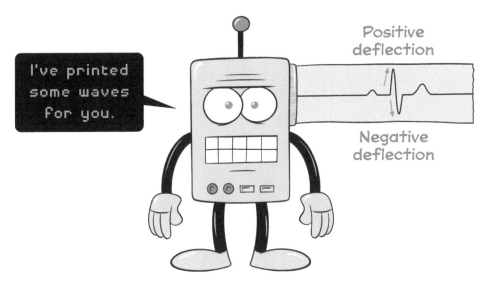

The vertical axis of the ECG is used to measure the height or depth of a wave, known as the wave's *amplitude*. It represents a measure of voltage in millivolts (mV). One small box represents 0.1 mV. In clinical practice, the amplitude of a wave (or elevation/depression of a segment) is usually referred to in millimeters.

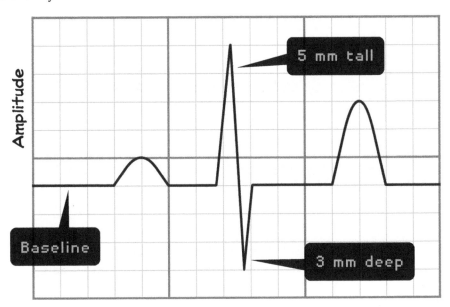

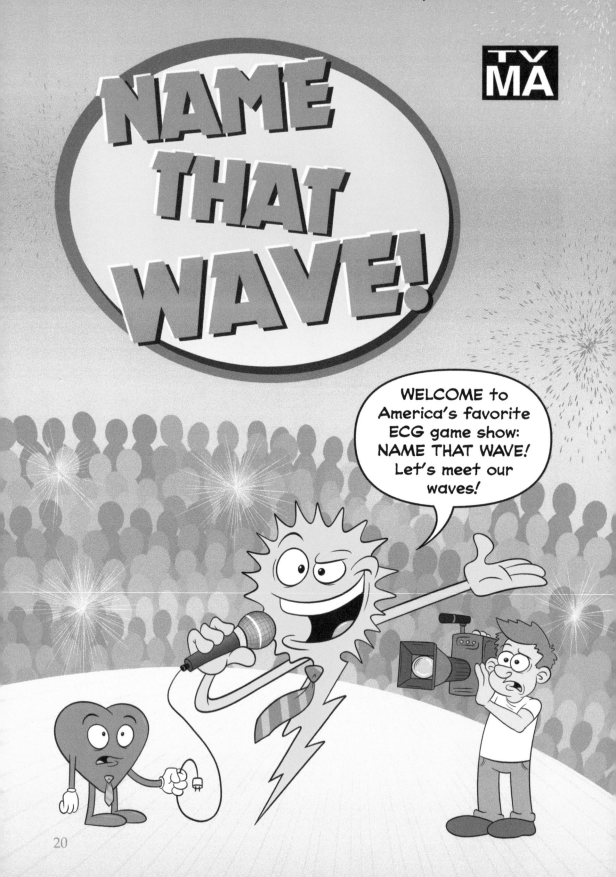

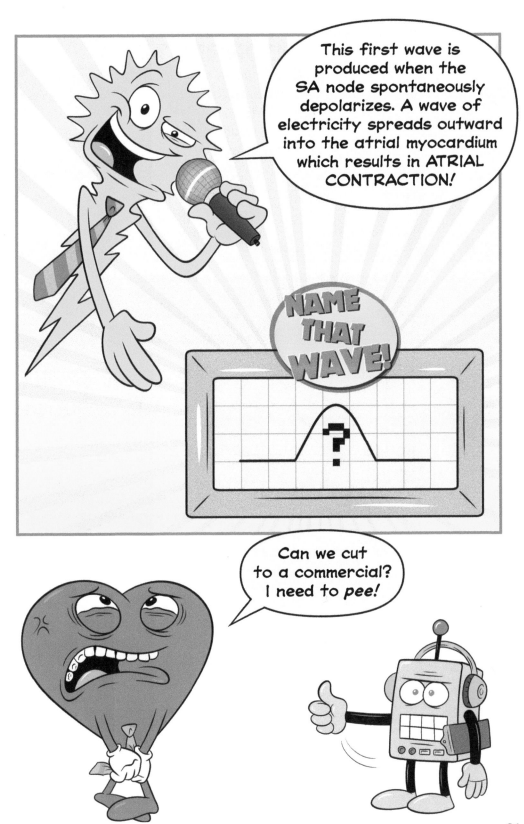

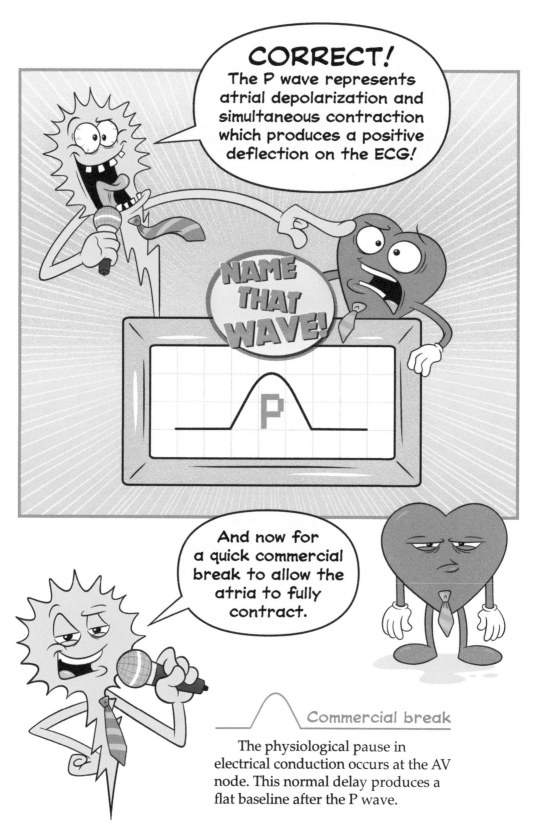

The physiological pause in electrical conduction occurs at the AV node. This normal delay produces a flat baseline after the P wave.

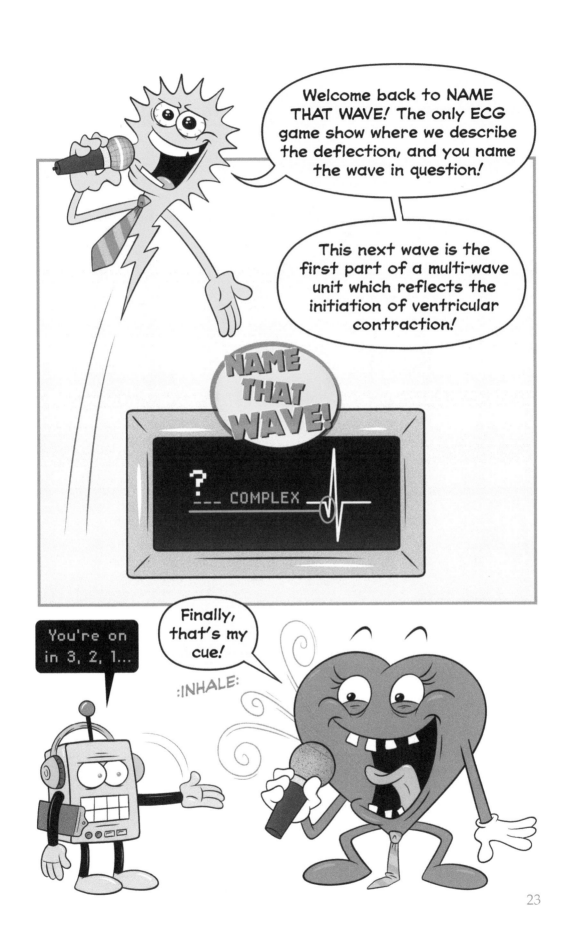

23

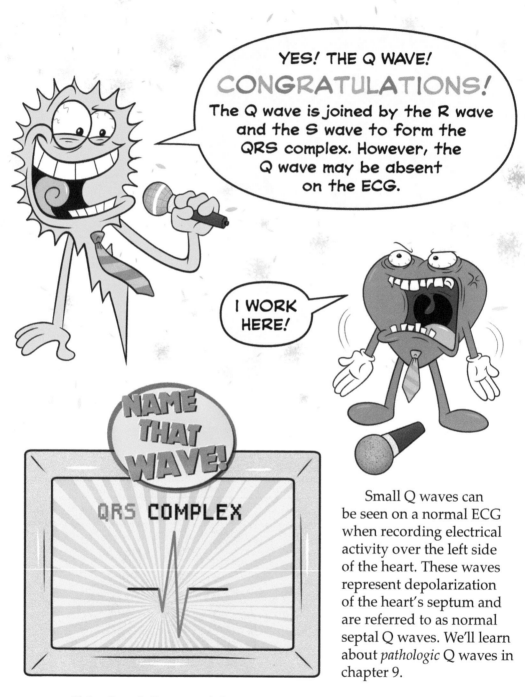

YES! THE Q WAVE! CONGRATULATIONS! The Q wave is joined by the R wave and the S wave to form the QRS complex. However, the Q wave may be absent on the ECG.

I WORK HERE!

NAME THAT WAVE!

QRS COMPLEX

Small Q waves can be seen on a normal ECG when recording electrical activity over the left side of the heart. These waves represent depolarization of the heart's septum and are referred to as normal septal Q waves. We'll learn about *pathologic* Q waves in chapter 9.

- If the first deflection of the QRS complex is downward, then it is called a Q wave.
- The first upward deflection of a QRS complex is called an R wave.
- Any downward deflection that follows an upward deflection is called an S wave.

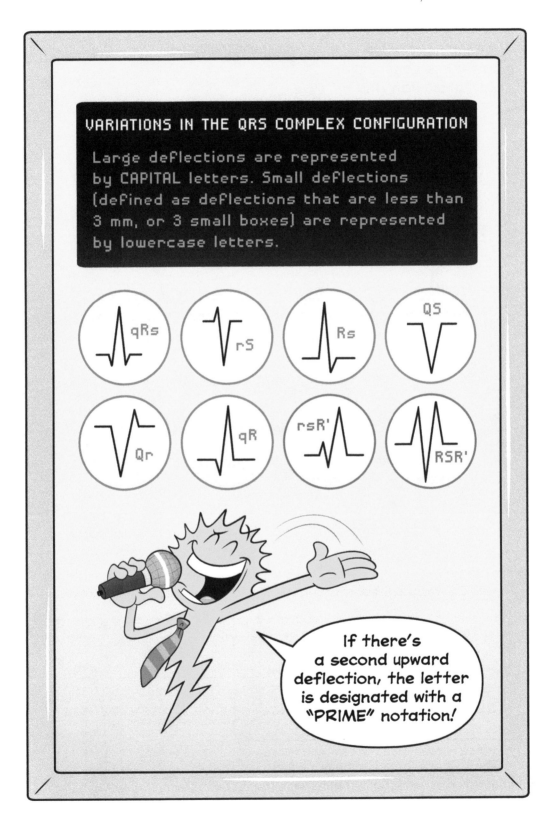

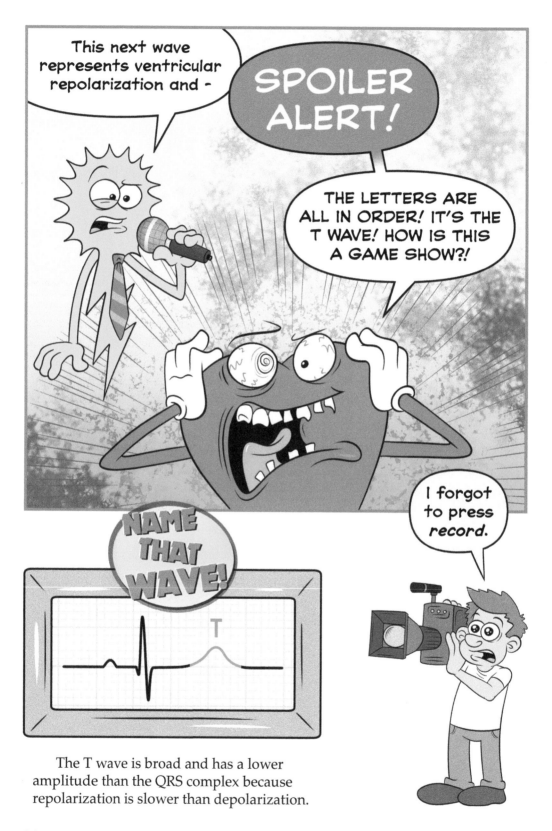

The T wave is broad and has a lower amplitude than the QRS complex because repolarization is slower than depolarization.

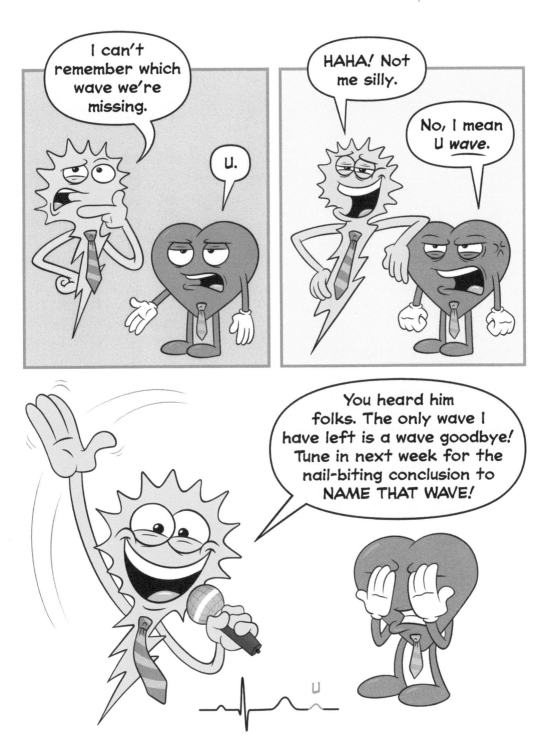

The U wave is not always present on the ECG. It typically appears as a small, upright deflection that follows the T wave. Its cause is unknown, but the U wave is thought to represent repolarization of the His-Purkinje system.

The ECG Waves

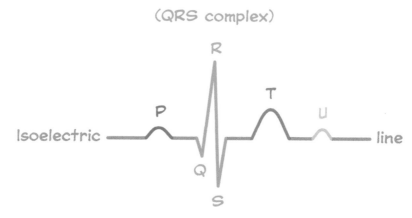

Let's take a closer look at the areas on the ECG that connect the waves together. These include the PR interval, the ST segment, and the QT interval. The baseline of the recording is also called the isoelectric line. In general terms, an *interval* describes an area on the ECG which includes a waveform plus a connecting straight line. A *segment* refers only to the line between two waves. Intervals and segments are named according to their beginning and endpoints with reference to the ECG waves.

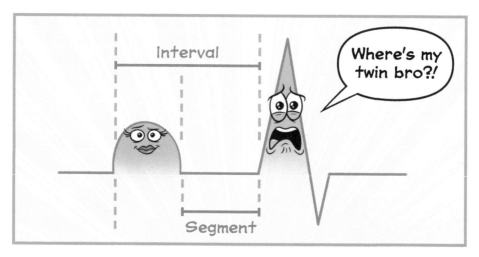

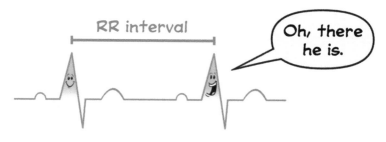

The RR interval is the area between two successive R waves.

The *PR interval* represents the time from the start of atrial depolarization to the start of ventricular depolarization. It is measured from the beginning of the P wave to the first part of the QRS complex. The PR interval includes the entire P wave as well as the line connecting it to the QRS complex. This connecting-line is called the PR segment.

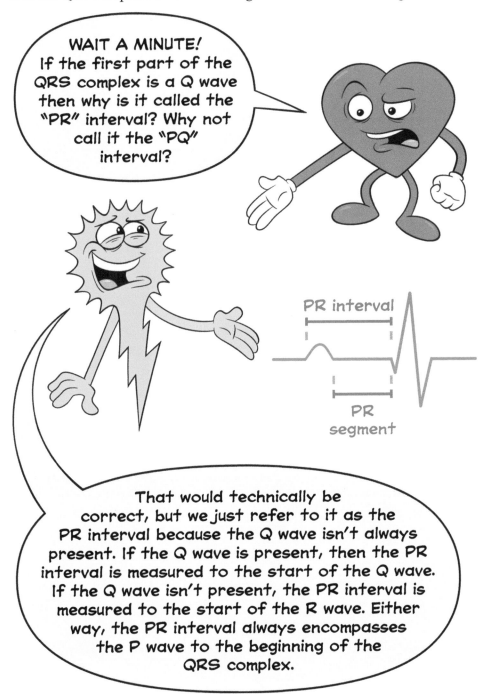

WAIT A MINUTE! If the first part of the QRS complex is a Q wave then why is it called the "PR" interval? Why not call it the "PQ" interval?

PR interval

PR segment

That would technically be correct, but we just refer to it as the PR interval because the Q wave isn't always present. If the Q wave is present, then the PR interval is measured to the start of the Q wave. If the Q wave isn't present, the PR interval is measured to the start of the R wave. Either way, the PR interval always encompasses the P wave to the beginning of the QRS complex.

The *ST segment* is a horizontal line which connects the end of the QRS complex to the beginning of the T wave. The ST segment represents the end of ventricular depolarization and the initiation of ventricular repolarization. The T wave itself represents a more rapid phase of repolarization. On a normal ECG the ST segment is level with other parts of the ECG's baseline.

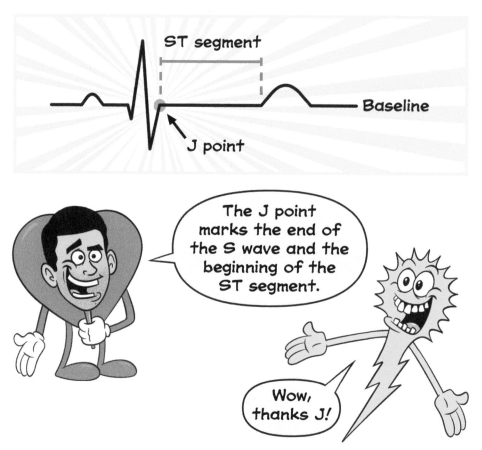

Elevation or depression of the ST segment beyond the ECG's baseline may be indicative of serious pathology such as myocardial ischemia or infarction.

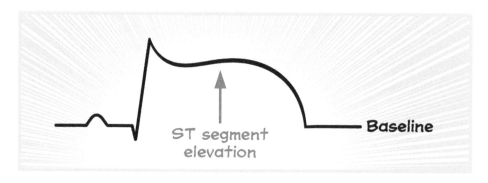

The *QT interval* represents the time taken for ventricular depolarization and repolarization. It's measured from the start of the QRS complex to the end of the T wave. The QT interval is inversely proportional to the heart rate. Therefore, a faster heart rate will produce a shorter QT interval while a slower heart rate will lengthen the QT interval.

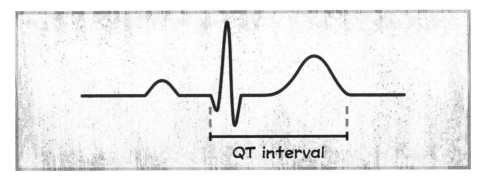

At normal sinus rates, the QT interval is considered normal when it's roughly less than half of the preceding RR interval. Due to the variability of the QT interval with the heart rate, a corrected QT interval, or QTc, is used to assess the absolute QT interval.

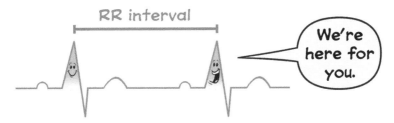

Bazett's formula is commonly used to calculate the corrected QT interval: the QTc is equal to the QT interval in seconds divided by the square root of the preceding RR interval in seconds. The normal value for the QTc varies with age and gender. The duration is slightly longer in females and increases slightly with age. The QTc is considered prolonged when it is greater than 0.44 seconds in males and 0.46 seconds in females.

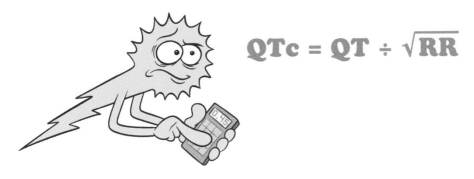

$$QTc = QT \div \sqrt{RR}$$

Conduction in Relation to the ECG

■ Depolarization   □ Repolarization

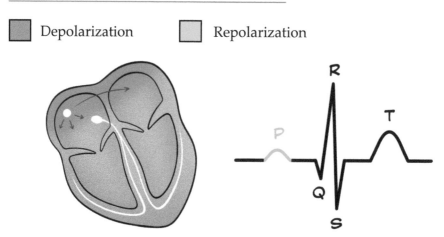

Atrial depolarization is initiated by the SA node, which causes the P wave.

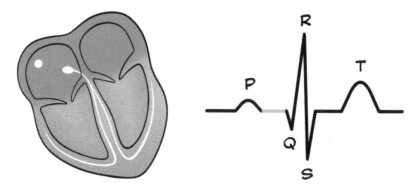

The wave of depolarization spreads completely throughout the atria and conduction is delayed at the AV node.

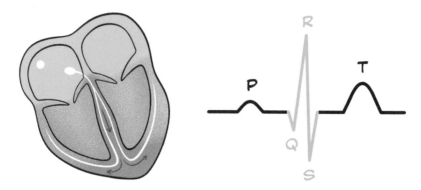

Atrial repolarization occurs as ventricular depolarization begins, which causes the QRS complex.

■ Depolarization   □ Repolarization

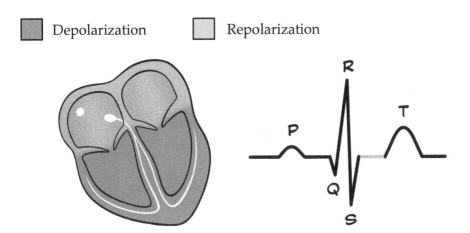

Ventricular depolarization is completed.

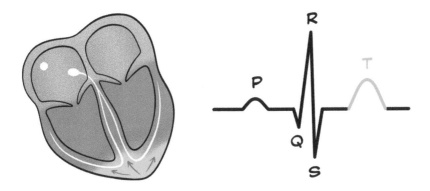

Ventricular repolarization spreads from the apex of the heart, which produces the T wave.

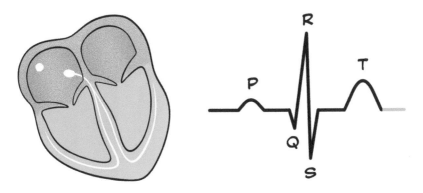

Ventricular repolarization is completed.

Introduction to Normal Values

- The duration of the **P wave** is normally less than 0.12 seconds (three small boxes). The amplitude is normally less than 2.5 mm in the limb leads and less than 1.5 mm in the precordial leads. A P wave normally precedes each QRS complex. The shape of the P wave is typically smooth and rounded.

- The duration of the **PR interval** is normally between 0.12 seconds to 0.20 seconds (three and five small boxes). The PR interval is normally isoelectric.

- The duration of the **Q wave** is normally less than 0.04 seconds (one small box).

- The duration of the **QRS complex** is also known as the QRS interval, which spans the Q wave, R wave, and S wave. It normally ranges from 0.07 to 0.11 seconds (less than three small boxes) and tends to be slightly longer in males than in females.

- The **ST segment** is typically flat and isoelectric, but slight deviations from the baseline may occur as normal variants. The most important cause of ST segment elevation is acute myocardial infarction.

- The **T wave** normally has an amplitude less than 5 mm in the limb leads and less than 15 mm in the precordial leads. The duration of the T wave is not usually measured because it is included in the calculation of the **QT interval** (see bottom of page 31).

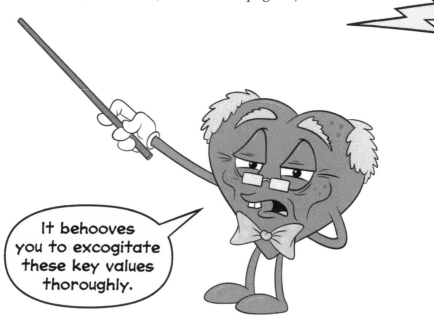

It behooves you to excogitate these key values thoroughly.

The amplitude of the QRS complex is typically greater than 5 mm in the limb leads and greater than 10 mm in the precordial leads. The upper limit of normal for the QRS amplitude can vary greatly.

Increased QRS amplitude (*high voltage*) may suggest the presence of left ventricular hypertrophy (LVH). The Sokolow-Lyon criteria are commonly used to to assess for evidence of LVH on the ECG. High voltage may also be a normal finding in young, athletic, or slim individuals.

Abnormally decreased QRS amplitude is known as *low voltage*. Some causes of low voltage include: pericardial effusion, pneumothorax, chronic obstructive pulmonary disease (COPD), obesity, infiltrative cardiomyopathy, constrictive pericarditis, and prior myocardial infarction.

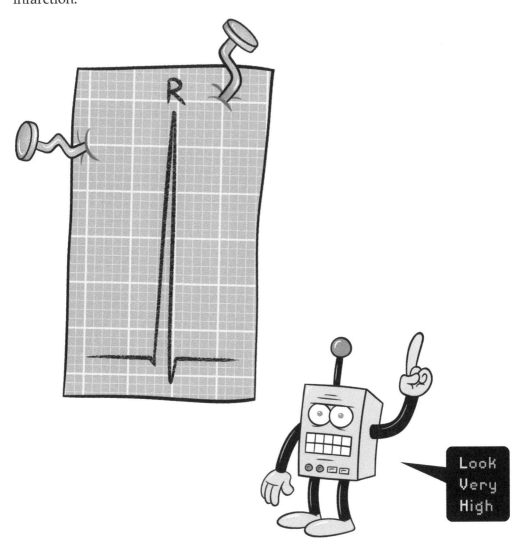

Sparkson's Summary: Chapter 2

- Each small box on an ECG represents a span of 0.04 seconds.

- Each large box consists of five small boxes and represents a span of 0.20 seconds.

- P wave: respresents atrial depolarization.

- QRS complex: represents ventricular depolarization.

- T wave: represents ventricular repolarization.

- U wave: may represent repolarization of the His-Purkinje system; not always present on the ECG.

- PR interval: measured from the start of the P wave to the beginning of the QRS complex.

- ST segment: connects the end of the QRS complex to the start of the T wave.

- QT interval: is measured from the start of the QRS complex to the end of the T wave. The corrected QT interval (QTc) is typically used in clinical practice.

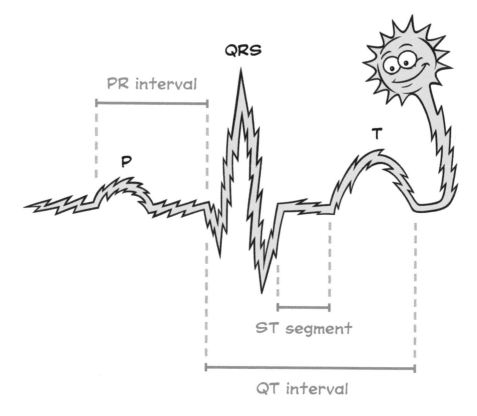

CHAPTER 3

RECORDING A 12-LEAD ECG

Electrodes and Leads

Electrodes are devices placed on the skin's surface in order to record the heart's electrical activity. The direction that the electric impulse travels relative to the electrode determines the wave's deflection on the ECG tracing.

During depolarization, an electric impulse that travels toward a positive electrode produces an upward deflection.

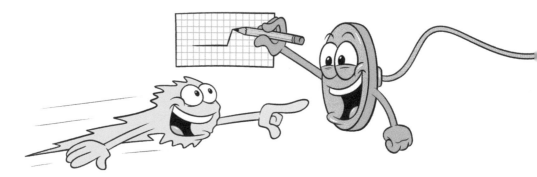

When the electric impulse travels away from a positive electrode a downward deflection is recorded.

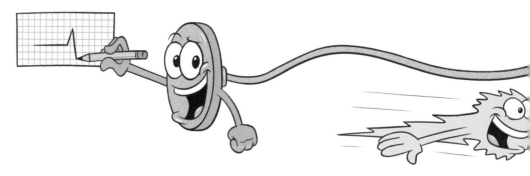

If the electric impulse travels perpendicularly to a positive electrode, then a biphasic wave is produced. A biphasic wave is part positive and part negative. If the wave is equally positive and negative, then the wave is termed equiphasic.

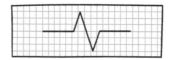

The effects of repolarization on a wave's deflection are the exact opposite of those depicted by depolarization in the illustrations above.

ECG tracings are generated with the placement of 10 electrodes on different areas of the body. A *lead* is a tracing of electrical activity between one positive pole and one negative pole. The standard ECG is composed of 12 separate leads, each of which provides a unique view of the heart's electrical activity.

Six limb leads are recorded by placing electrodes on the arms and legs. The other six leads are called *precordial leads* and are obtained by placing six electrodes across the chest. The precordial leads are also commonly referred to as *chest lead*s.

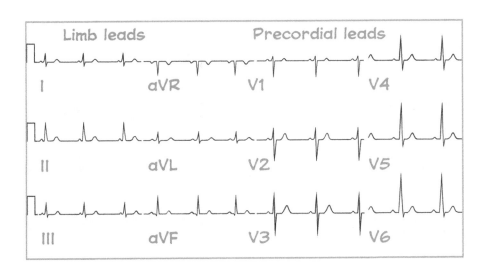

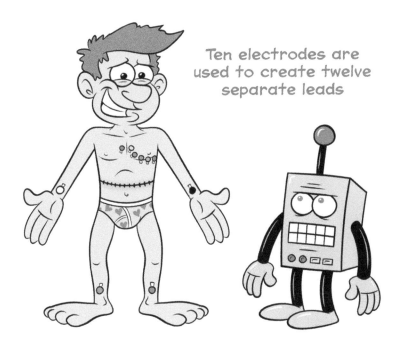

Ten electrodes are used to create twelve separate leads

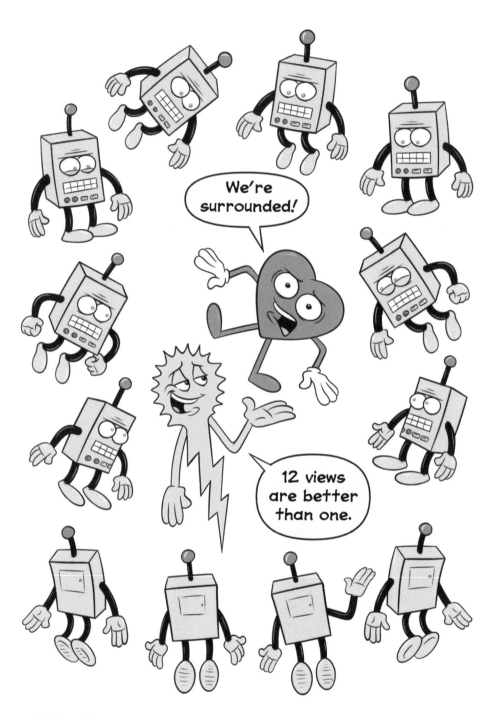

We're able to extract as much information as possible from an ECG recording by looking at the heart's electrical activity from a variety of different angles. A wave that is difficult to interpret on any given lead might be better visualized at another lead, which represents an alternative viewpoint of the same electrical activity.

The six limb leads are grouped into three bipolar leads and three augmented (unipolar) leads. The limb leads offer a view of the heart's frontal plane, which lies on an imaginary vertical cross-section of the heart.

The six precordial leads are unipolar leads and provide a view of the heart's horizontal plane, which lies on an imaginary transverse cross-section of the heart.

Planes

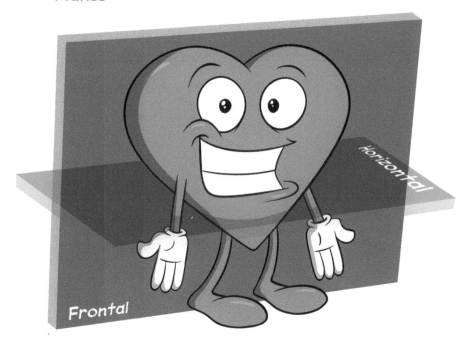

Limb leads lie on the frontal plane

Precordial leads lie on the horizontal plane

Bipolar leads use a positive and negative electrode to produce an ECG tracing. They also use a third ground electrode which helps prevent electrical interference from appearing on the recording. The bipolar leads consist of limb leads I, II, and III.

Unipolar leads require only a positive electrode. These include the three augmented limb leads aVR, aVL, and aVF, as well as the six precordial leads (V1 through V6).

The ECG machine is able to make any skin electrode positive or negative in order to produce the different limb leads.

The Bipolar Limb Leads (I, II, III)

Lead I is created by making the electrode on the left arm positive and the electrode on the right arm negative. Electrical current flows towards the positive electrode and away from the negative electrode. Therefore, lead I provides us with a left lateral view of the heart.

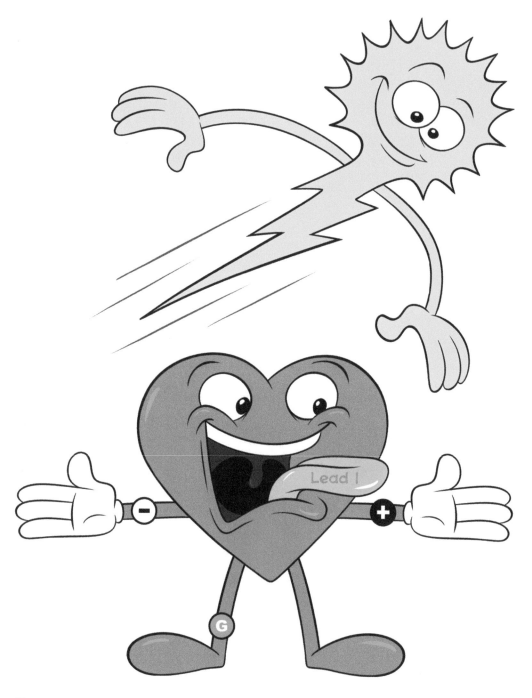

Lead II is created by making the electrode on the left leg positive and the electrode on the right arm negative. Lead II gives us a view of the inferior heart wall.

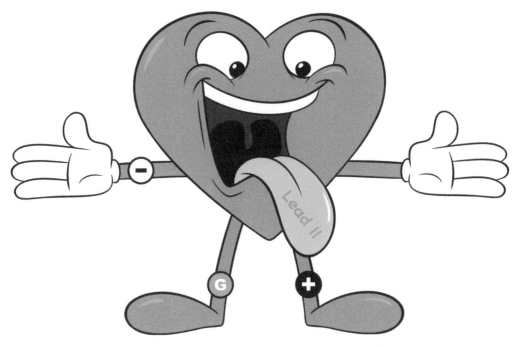

Lead III is created by making the electrode on the left leg positive and the electrode on the left arm negative. Lead III also provides an inferior view of the heart.

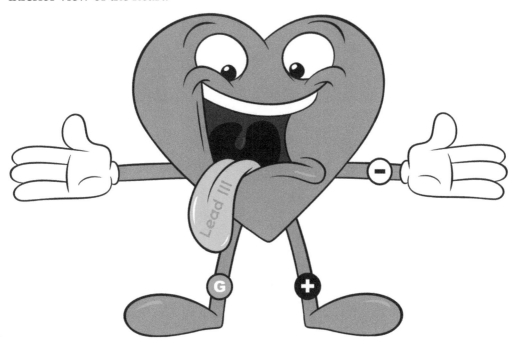

Einthoven's Triangle

The bipolar limb lead configuration is also known as *Einthoven's triangle,* named after the Dutch physiologist, Dr. Willem Einthoven. Einthoven pioneered the ECG and won the Nobel prize in medicine in 1924 for his work.

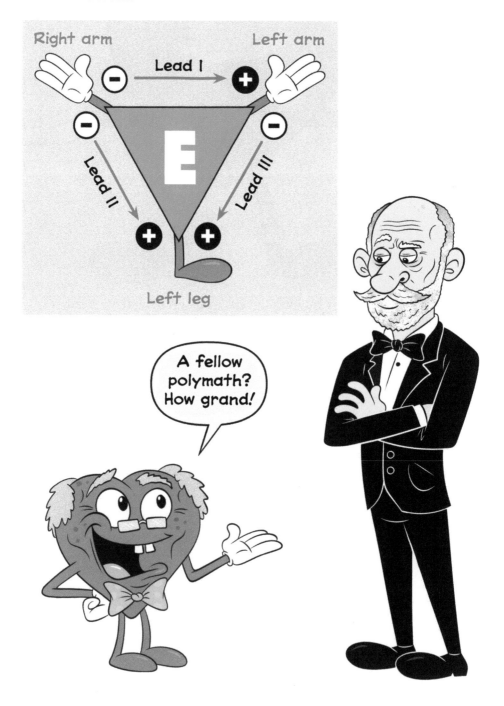

The Augmented Limb Leads (aVR, aVL, aVF)

These unipolar leads are called augmented leads because the ECG machine must amplify the voltage in order to get adequate recordings.

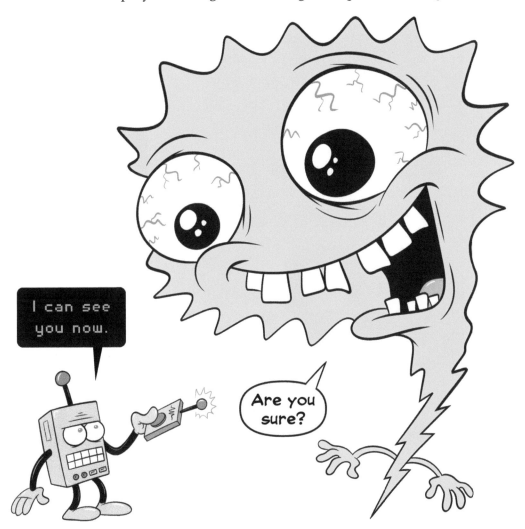

Lead aVR (Augmented Voltage Right) is created by making the electrode on the right arm positive. The electrodes on the left arm and left leg serve as a common ground and are both negative.

Lead aVL (Augmented Voltage Left) is created by making the electrode on the left arm positive. The electrodes on the right arm and left leg serve as a common ground and are both negative.

Lead aVF (augmented Voltage Foot) is created by making the electrode of the leg positive. The electrodes of the left and right arms serve as a common ground and are both negative.

Lead aVR provides a view of the right upper side of the heart.

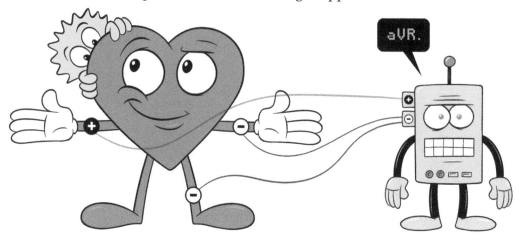

Lead aVL provides a view of the left lateral heart wall.

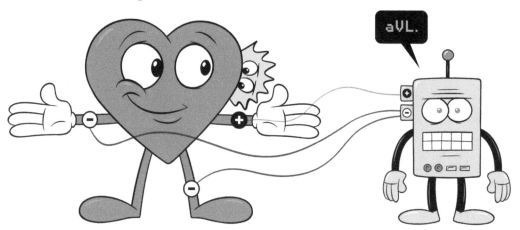

Lead aVF provides a view of the inferior heart wall.

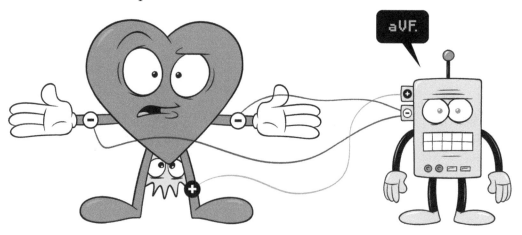

The Precordial Leads (V1-V6)

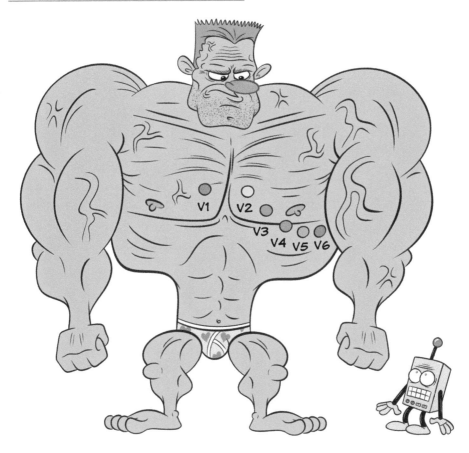

The six precordial (chest) leads are created by placing six positive electrodes across the chest. The electrodes are numbered in order beginning from the right side of the chest towards the left side. The precordial leads provide a view of the heart's electrical activity on the horizontal plane.

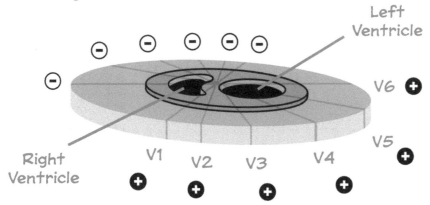

Generating the Precordial Leads

Accurate placement of chest electrodes is necessary in order to produce reliable precordial leads.

- Lead V1 requires placement of a positive electrode in the fourth intercostal space to the right of the sternum.

- Lead V2 requires placement of a positive electrode in the fourth intercostal space to the left of the sternum.

- Leads V3 requires placement of a positive electrode between the electrodes for V2 and V4. It often helps to place the electrode for V4 first and then go back to place the electrode for V3.

- Lead V4 requires placement of a positive electrode in the fifth intercostal space at the midclavicular line (MCL).

- Lead V5 requires placement of a positive electrode between the electrodes for V4 and V6.

- Lead V6 requires placement of a positive electrode in the fifth intercostal space at the midaxillary line (MAL).

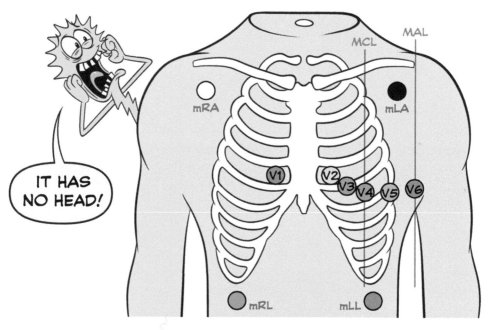

The limb electrodes can be placed in modified positions so that all the leads are obtained from electrodes on the trunk. These electrodes are designated as the *modified right arm electrode* (mRA), *modified left arm electrode* (mLA), *modified right leg electrode* (mRL), and *modified left leg electrode* (mLL). This technique is useful in the setting of prehospital care and certain circumstances within the hospital environment.

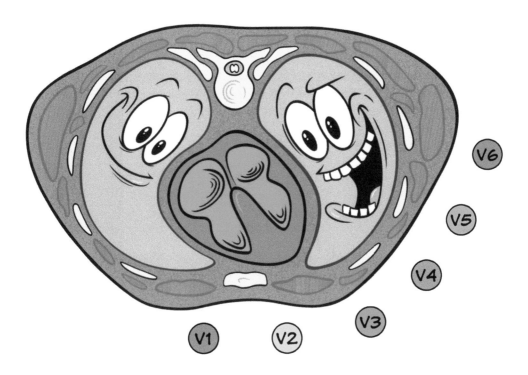

Each chest lead provides a unique line of site through the heart. Leads V1 and V2 are oriented to provide a view of the septum. Leads V3 and V4 are oriented over the anterior aspect of the heart. Leads V5 and V6 are oriented over the lateral aspect of the left ventricle. Limb leads I and aVL join V5 and V6 to complete the left lateral lead group. Technically, there is some overlap in the lead groupings, as lead V2 is both septal and anterior, and lead V4 is both anterior and lateral.

Summary of lead groups:

Septal	Anterior	Lateral	Inferior
V1	V3	V5	II
V2	V4	V6	III
		I	aVF
		aVL	

Anatomy of the Electrocardiogram

A standard ECG printout displays its 12 leads in a standard order. Lead markers and lead names organize the ECG into sections. A standardization mark is typically 10 small boxes in height and calibrates the ECG tracking. At the bottom of the printout we can usually find a 10 second rhythm strip, which is often generated from lead II.

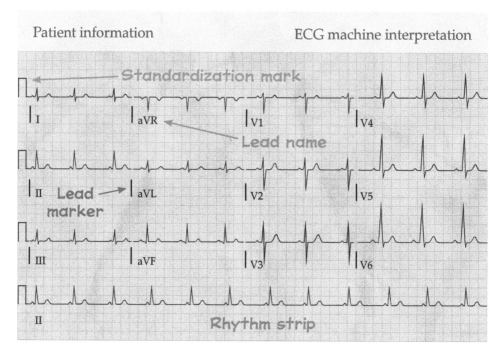

A record of the heart's electrical activity can be obtained from a variety of ECG machines. Some provide a complete 12-lead printout, while others simply provide an extended rhythm strip. Some devices can also be used for continuous cardiac monitoring, in which the heart's electrical activity is observable from a live display.

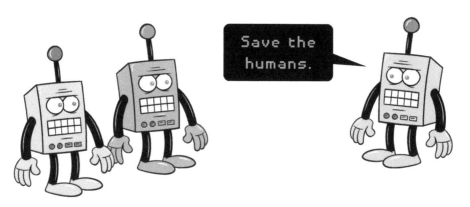

ECG Limitations

Human error should be considered as a potential source of electrocardiographic abnormalities. An unreliable ECG may be caused by electrode reversal, electrode misplacement, wire disconnection, and artifact. These abnormalities have recognizable patterns on the ECG which help distinguish them from true pathology.

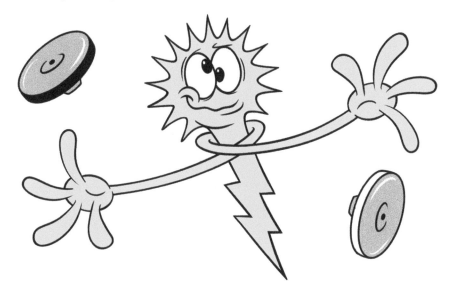

Reversal of left arm and right arm electrodes

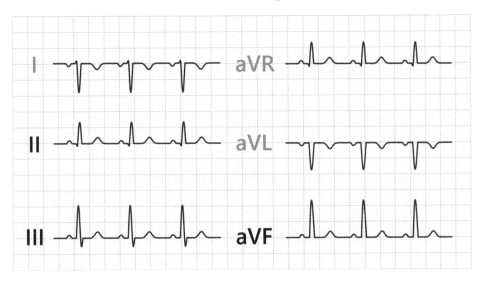

Mixing up the left arm and right arm electrodes is a common error that causes leads I and aVL to become inverted and lead aVR to become positive. This ECG pattern is similarly seen in the setting of dextrocardia.

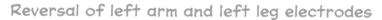

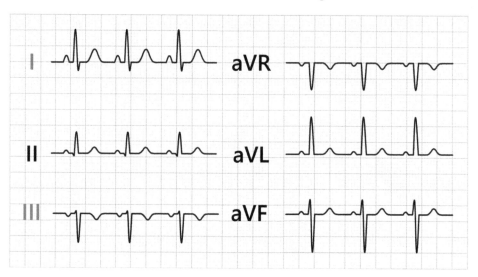

If the left arm and left leg electrodes are switched then the amplitude of the P wave in lead I may be unexpectedly greater than the P wave in lead II. The reversal also causes lead III to become inverted.

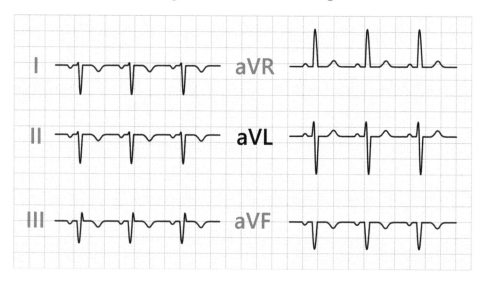

Reversal of the right arm and left leg electrodes causes inversions in leads I, II, III, and aVF. Lead aVR becomes positive.

The ground electrode is usually placed on the right leg and helps prevent electrical interference from appearing on the ECG. Reversal of the right leg and either arm electrode results in very low amplitudes in an isolated limb lead. Right leg and right arm electrode reversal produces a near flat line in lead II, while right leg and left arm electrode reversal produces a near flatline in lead III.

Reversal of the precordial electrodes disturbs the normal R wave progression in the chest leads. For example, a predominant R wave may be seen in lead V1.

Normal R wave progression from V1 to V6

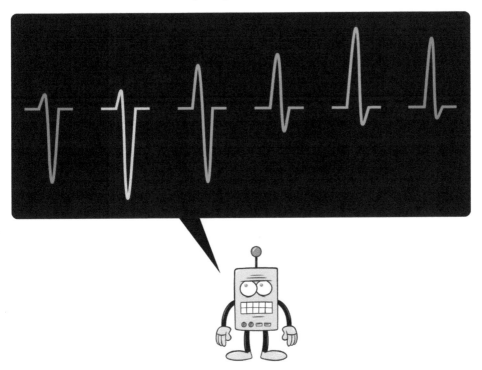

The electrodes need to placed in the correct order to avoid lead reversal. They also need to be placed accurately according to anatomic landmarks. In women, the precordial electrodes should be placed under the left breast to ensure a reliable ECG tracing.

Another source of error to consider is *artifact*, which refers to ECG abnormalities caused by movement from the patient or outside electrical interference.

History and Physical

The ECG should be interpreted in the context of the clinical scenario in which it is obtained. A thorough understanding of a patient's clinical history and chief complaint will affect your pretest probabilities for different diagnoses. Consider the patient's:

- History of present illness

- Age, gender, race, occupation, reliability of historian

- Vital signs: height, weight, BMI, blood pressure, temperature, pulse, respirations

- Past medical history: cardiovascular, endocrine, pulmonary, renal, infectious disease, hematologic, oncologic, rheumatologic, etc.

- Family history: coronary artery disease, sudden cardiac death, cardiac devices, etc.

- Social history: tobacco use, illicit drug use, alcohol consumption

- History of surgeries, port placements, or dialysis access

- Recent hospitalizations

- Medications

- Allergies

- Review of systems

- Physical exam

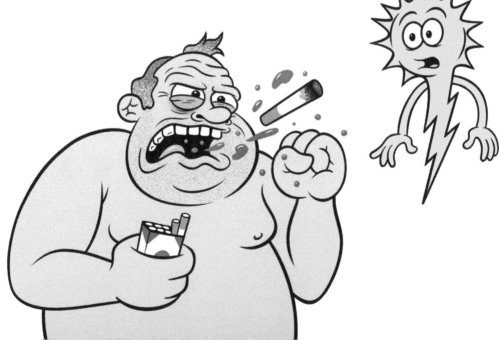

Approach to ECG Interpretation

It's important to establish a systematic method when reading a 12-lead ECG. Following a standardized sequence of steps helps us avoid overlooking abnormalities on the ECG tracing which may be of critical clinical significance. We'll review the details of each of these steps in the chapters that follow.

1. Rate
2. Rhythm
   a. Assess regularity
   b. Check the P waves
   c. Determine the QRS duration
   d. Determine the intervals (PR, QT)
3. Axis
4. Hypertrophy
5. Infarction

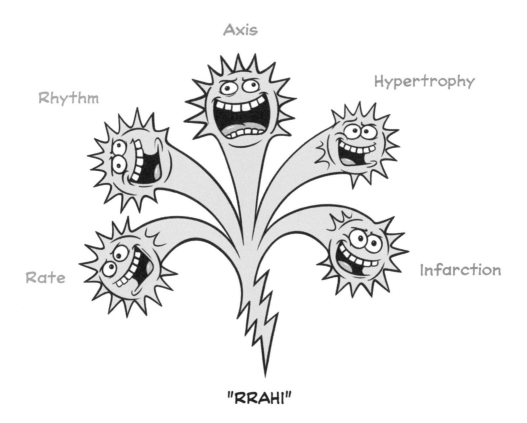

"RRAHI"

Sparkson's Summary: Chapter 3

- A 12-lead ECG consists of six limb leads (I, II, III, aVR, aVL, aVF) and six precordial leads (V1, V2, V3, V4, V5, V6).

- Inferior leads: II, III, aVF

- Lateral leads: I, aVL, V5, V6

- Septal leads: V1, V2

- Anterior leads: V3, V4

- The limb leads provide a view of the heart's electrical activity on the frontal plane.

- The precordial leads provide a view of the heart's electrical activity on the horizontal plane.

- Electrocardiographic abnormalities may be benign or represent pathology. They can also be caused by electrode reversal, electrode misplacement, wire disconnection, and artifact.

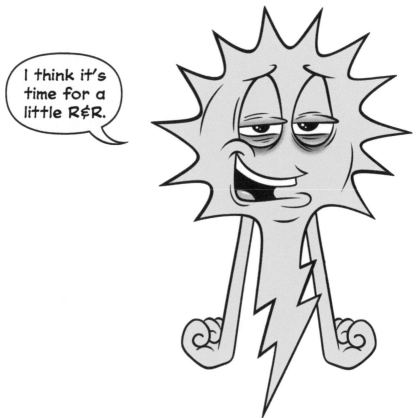

I think it's time for a little R&R.

CHAPTER 4

RATE AND RHYTHM

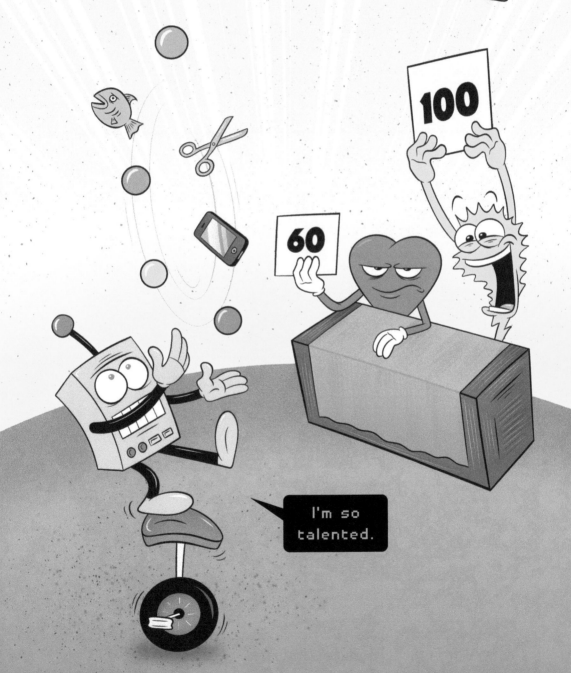

Rate

The first step in ECG interpretation is determining the rate. We describe the heart rate as the number of beats per minute. There are several different methods to calculate the rate including the counting method, the 6-second method, and the 1500 method. The ECG machine usually includes its own calculation of the rate at the top of the printout, but in certain cases this reading may be inaccurate.

Recall that one small box on an ECG strip equals 0.04 seconds, and one large box (composed of 5x5 small boxes) equals 0.2 seconds. Therefore, a span of five large boxes represents one second.

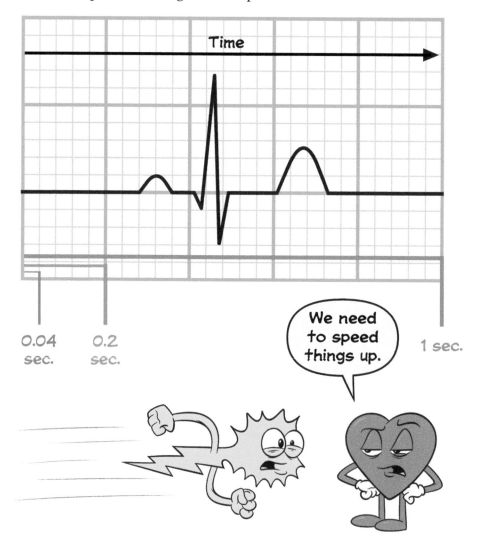

A cardiac cycle that repeats itself once every five large boxes (a span of one second) would result in a heart rate of 60 beats per minute.

The heart's dominant pacemaker and center of automaticity is the SA node (also known as the sinus node). It maintains normal sinus rhythm (NSR) at a rate between 60 and 100 beats per minute.

The number within this range can vary depending on inputs to the SA node from the autonomic nervous system.

Normal sinus rhythm

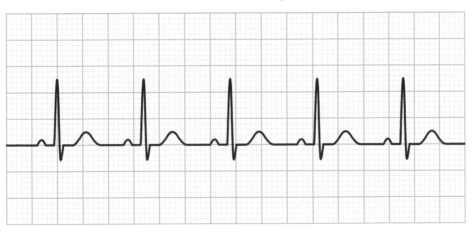

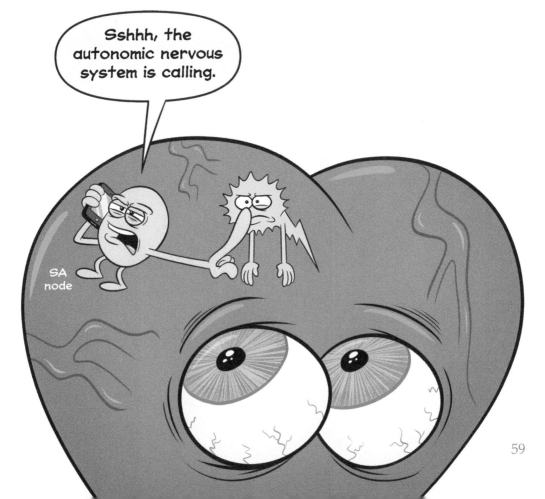

The Autonomic Nervous System

The peripheral nervous system is the part of nervous system located outside of the central nervous system. Within the peripheral nervous system lies the autonomic nervous system (ANS), also known as the involuntary nervous system.

The ANS consists of motor neurons that regulate the activity of glands, smooth muscle, and (most importantly for this book) cardiac muscle. It has two subdivisions, the sympathetic and parasympathetic divisions. These two divisions work in opposition to each other – the sympathetic division stimulates the heart while the parasympathetic division inhibits it.

Sympathetic: fight or flight

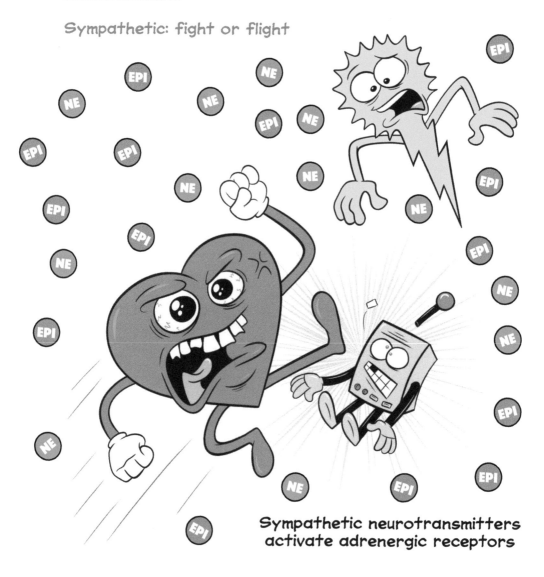

Sympathetic neurotransmitters activate adrenergic receptors

The sympathetic nervous system releases neurotransmitters called catecholamines [epinephrine (EPI) and norepinephrine (NE)] that markedly increase the activity of the heart. These cardiac excitatory effects include an increase in the rate of SA node pacing (positive chronotropic effect), enhanced force of contraction of the heart muscle (positive inotropic effect), and an acceleration of atrioventricular electrical conduction (positive dromotropic effect).

The parasympathetic nervous system releases the neurotransmitter acetylcholine (ACh), which produces opposite effects on the heart (negative chronotropic, inotropic, and dromotropic effects).

Parasympathetic: rest and digest

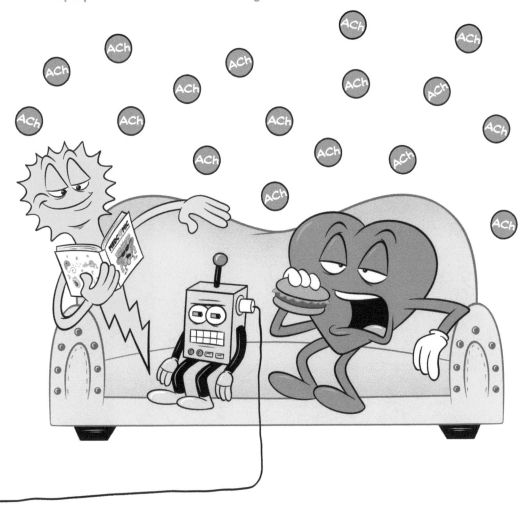

Parasympathetic neurotransmitters activate cholinergic receptors

Sinus bradycardia is a rhythm that occurs when the SA node produces impulses at a rate slower than 60 times per minute.

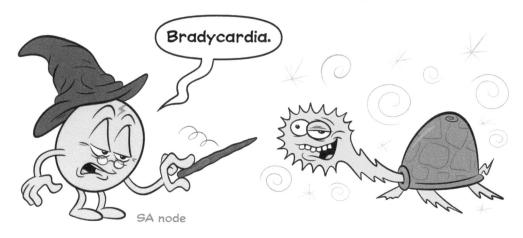

Sinus tachycardia is a rhythm that occurs when the SA node produces impulses at a rate faster than 100 times per minute.

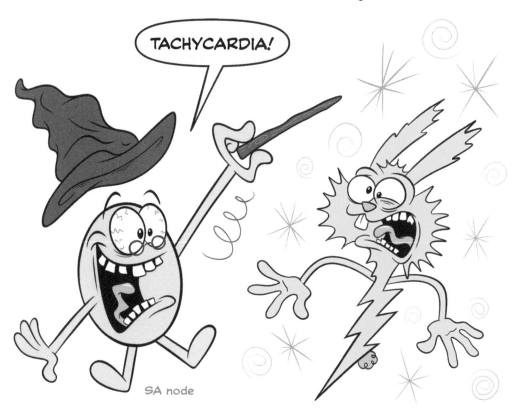

Both sinus bradycardia and sinus tachycardia can occur due to the effects of drugs or varying inputs from the autonomic nervous system. We'll discuss these two rhythms in greater detail in chapter 7.

Ectopic Foci

Ectopic foci are potential pacemaker sites within the heart located outside of the SA node. The term "ectopic foci" refers to a group of potential pacemakers, while the term "ectopic focus" refers to a singular site. Like the SA node, ectopic foci display automaticity, or the ability to spontaneously depolarize. However, their pacemaking ability is usually suppressed by the faster rate of the dominant SA node. This is a key concept - the higher frequency of depolarization from the dominant pacemaking site suppresses all other slower potential pacemakers by a mechanism called *overdrive suppression*.

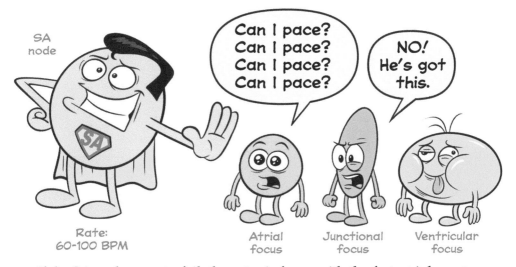

If the SA node were to fail, the ectopic focus with the fastest inherent rate of depolarization assumes responsibility for pacemaking activity and suppresses all the slower ectopic foci below it. If the ectopic focus sustains the rhythm, the overall rhythm is known as an *ectopic rhythm*. This heroic fail-safe system saves lives.

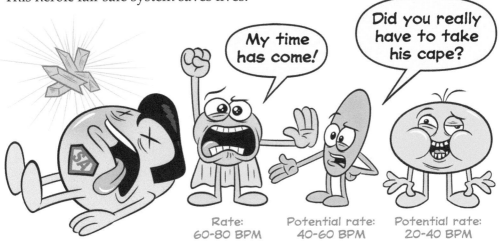

Levels of Ectopic Foci

Potential pacemakers can be found at different levels of the heart, each with their own inherent rate of pacing.

- **Atrial foci**: potential pacemakers at the level of the atria have an inherent pacing rate of 60 to 80 beats per minute.
- **Junctional foci**: potential pacemakers at the level of the AV junction have an inherent pacing rate of 40 to 60 beats per minute.
- **Ventricular foci**: potential pacemakers at the level of the ventricles have an inherent pacing rate of 20 to 40 beats per minute.

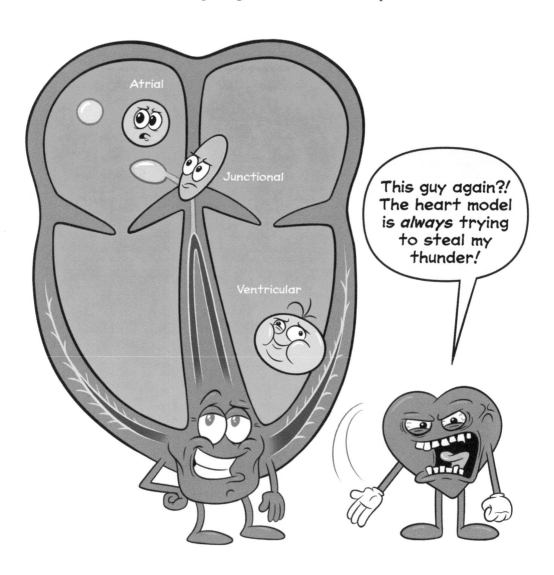

Ectopic foci within the atria produce P waves with a unique shape compared to a normal sinus P wave. These abnormal P waves are called P' (pronounced "P-prime") waves.

The transfer of pacing responsibility occurs in a specific order. This order depends on the inherent rate of depolarization for each level of foci, which decreases at each level.

If the SA node fails, the foci at the level of the atria will begin pacing at a rate of 60 to 80 beats per minute.

If the atrial foci fail, the foci at the level of the atrioventricular junction will begin pacing at a rate of 40 to 60 beats per minute.

If the junctional foci fail, the foci at the level of the ventricles will begin pacing at a rate of 20 to 40 beats per minute.

If the ventricular foci fail there is a high risk of deterioration to -

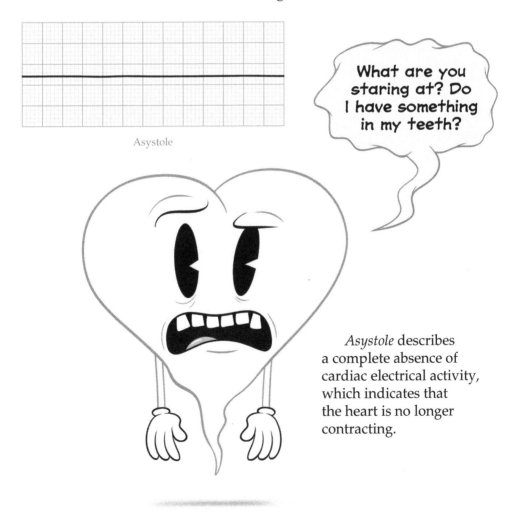

Asystole

What are you staring at? Do I have something in my teeth?

Asystole describes a complete absence of cardiac electrical activity, which indicates that the heart is no longer contracting.

The Counting Method

This method is ideal for calculating regular heart rates.

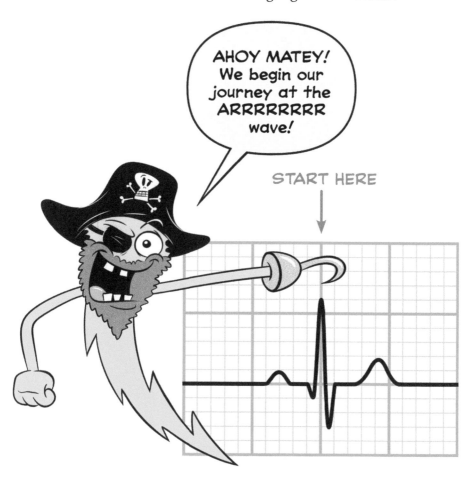

Look for an R wave on the ECG tracing that lands on a dark vertical line. Calculating the rate begins here.

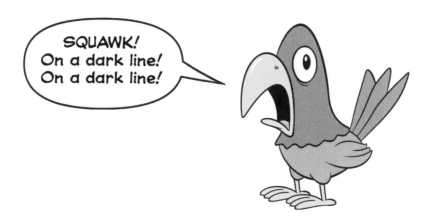

Each dark line *after* the line we started on will be named according to the following list of numbers, which should be memorized in order:

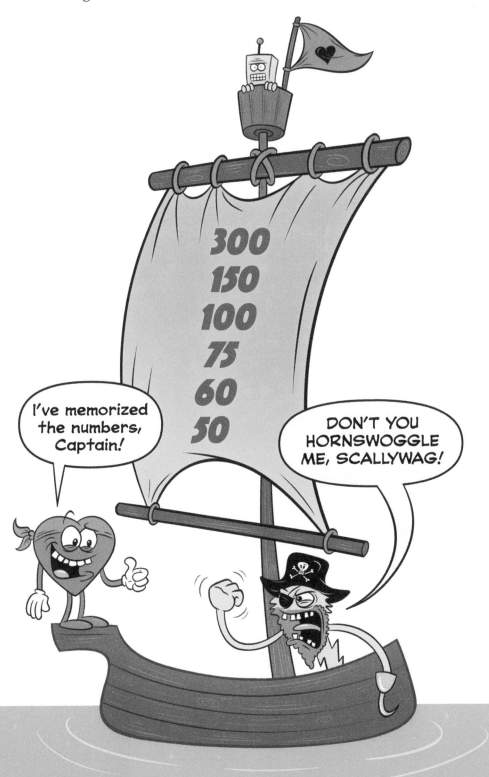

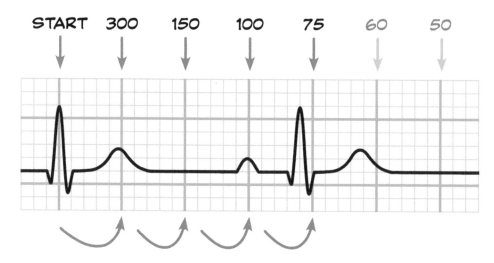

Count off the list of numbers for each dark line after the start point. The heart rate is determined by the next R wave. As you can see in the example above, the next R wave appears between 75 and 100, which is normal. We'll estimate the heart rate to be about 79 beats per minute. The other numbers were listed in the diagram, but we didn't need to count them off in this case.

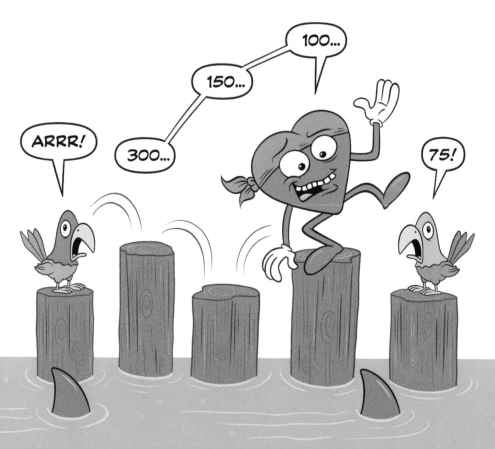

Let's practice! Determine the rate for each strip below.

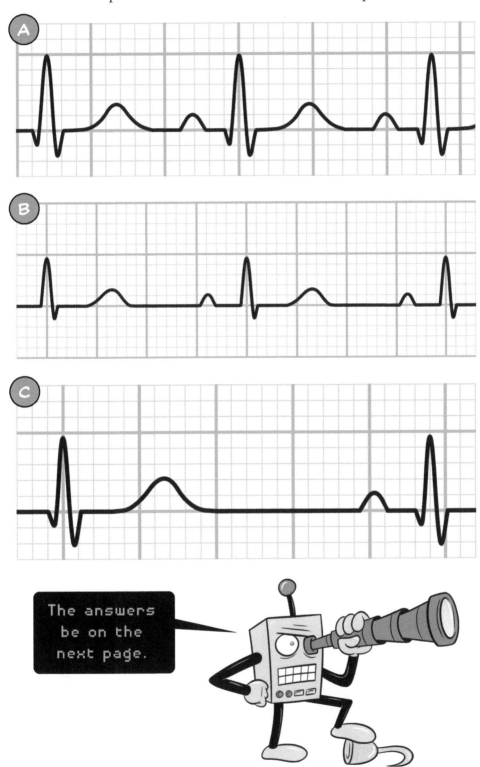

The answers be on the next page.

Answers:

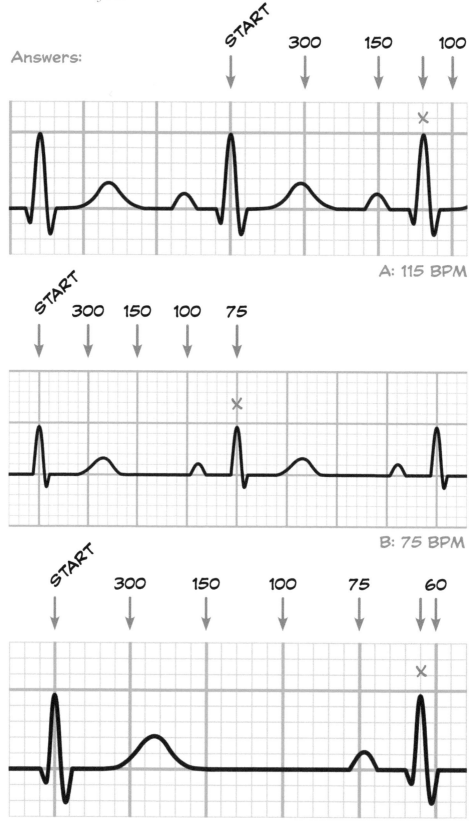

A: 115 BPM

B: 75 BPM

C: 62 BPM

Further precision can be obtained by assigning rate values to the thin lines on the ECG. It is not necessary to commit these values to memory. Using the identified values for the thin lines is useful in the counting method when the second R wave lies between two dark lines.

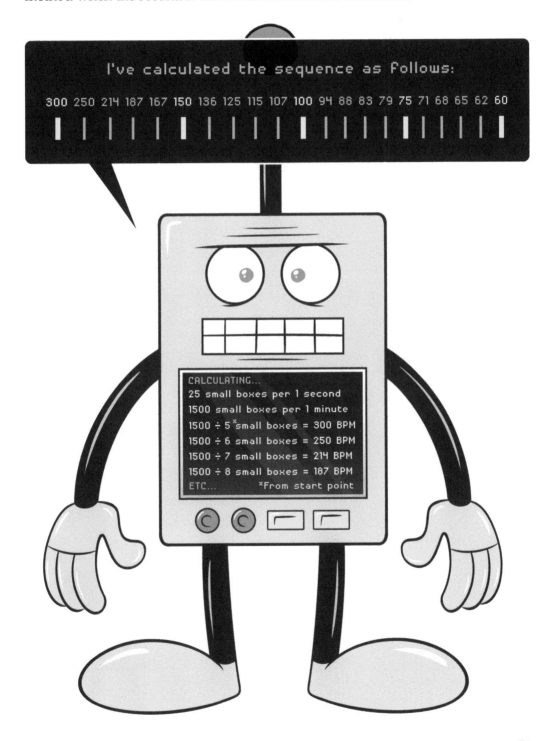

I've calculated the sequence as follows:

300 250 214 187 167 150 136 125 115 107 100 94 88 83 79 75 71 68 65 62 60

CALCULATING...
25 small boxes per 1 second
1500 small boxes per 1 minute
1500 ÷ 5*small boxes = 300 BPM
1500 ÷ 6 small boxes = 250 BPM
1500 ÷ 7 small boxes = 214 BPM
1500 ÷ 8 small boxes = 187 BPM
ETC...   *From start point

The 6-second Method

The 6-second method is useful for slow or irregular rhythms. A span of 15 large boxes represents a duration of 3 seconds (0.20 sec. x 15). For convenience, most ECG rhythm strips mark off 3 second intervals along the upper margin of the graph paper. Single-lead ECG rhythm strips are often printed from ECG monitors in critical care areas of the hospital. The rhythm strip can be as long as needed and helps to identify any sudden abnormal electrical activity.

Using the 3 second marks on the ECG rhythm strip allows us to quickly calculate the rate in a 6 second period. Count the number of QRS complexes within the 6 second interval and multiply that number by 10. This gives you an estimate of the rate. That's it!

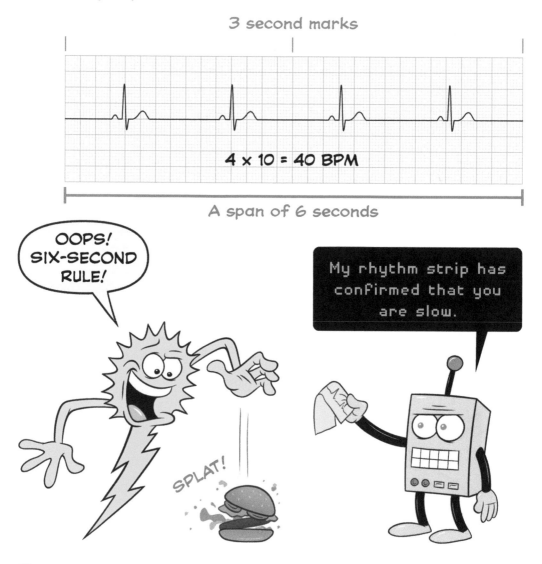

3 second marks

4 x 10 = 40 BPM

A span of 6 seconds

OOPS! SIX-SECOND RULE!

SPLAT!

My rhythm strip has confirmed that you are slow.

The 1500 Method

The 1500 method is an accurate technique to calculate the rate, but cannot be used for irregular rhythms. To use the 1500 method, count the number of small boxes between two consecutive R waves and divide 1500 by that number.

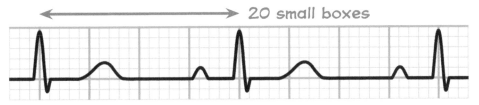

20 small boxes

1500 divided by 20 small boxes = 75 beats per minute

Normal Heart Rates in Children

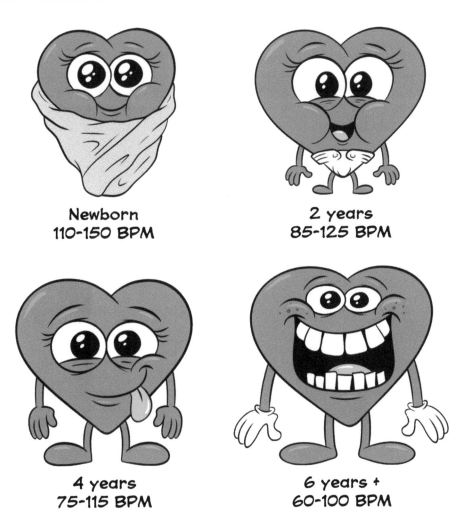

Newborn
110-150 BPM

2 years
85-125 BPM

4 years
75-115 BPM

6 years +
60-100 BPM

Rhythm

After determining the rate, we should evaluate the rhythm. While rate refers to the frequency of the heart in beats per minute, *rhythm* refers to the pattern. An ECG with a *regular* rhythm has equal R to R intervals throughout the tracing. Otherwise, the rhythm is described to be irregular. Normal sinus rhythm, sinus bradycardia, and sinus tachycardia all have regular rhythms because they remain on beat like a metronome.

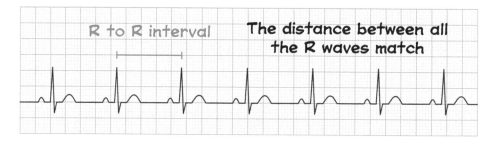

The term *arrhythmia* is used to denote any abnormal rhythm. Arrhythmia literally means "an absence of rhythm." Some would argue that the term *dysrhythmia* is more accurate, which means "bad rhythm." In general, these terms may be used interchangeably in reference to any abnormal rhythm.

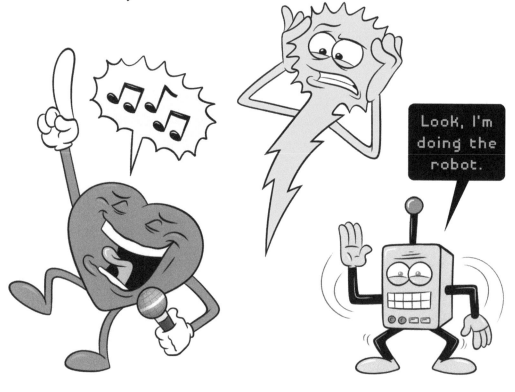

To perform a proper rhythm interpretation we need to evaluate the major components of the ECG tracing. After assessing for regularity, look for P waves and determine whether they are regular or not. If P waves are absent, we can infer that an ectopic focus is generating the rhythm below the atria, at the level of the AV junction or ventricles. If P waves are present, then we need to check if they are normal and identical to each other.

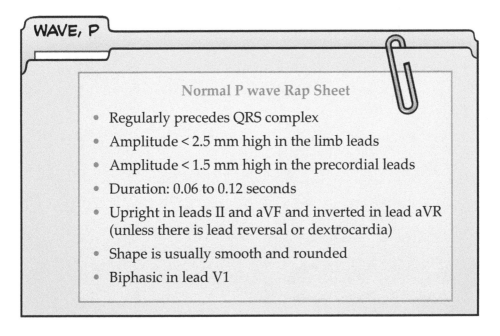

WAVE, P

Normal P wave Rap Sheet

- Regularly precedes QRS complex
- Amplitude < 2.5 mm high in the limb leads
- Amplitude < 1.5 mm high in the precordial leads
- Duration: 0.06 to 0.12 seconds
- Upright in leads II and aVF and inverted in lead aVR (unless there is lead reversal or dextrocardia)
- Shape is usually smooth and rounded
- Biphasic in lead V1

P waves and QRS complexes normally correlate in a one to one fashion. However, this correlation can be disrupted when the atria and ventricles are under the control of separate pacemakers and beat independently of each other. This abnormality is called *AV dissociation*.

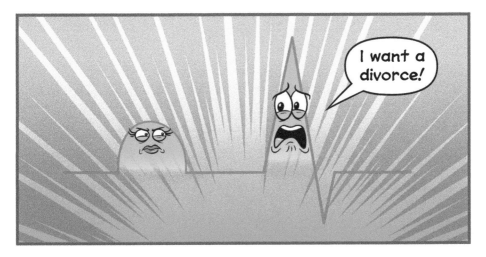

It is also important to assess the duration of the QRS complex. A normal QRS complex spans 0.04 to 0.12 seconds, or 1 to 3 small boxes. As you review the ECG tracing, ask yourself whether the QRS complexes are narrow or wide.

Next, determine the PR interval. Recall that a normal PR interval is 0.12 to 0.20 seconds long, or 3 to 5 small boxes.

Normal Sinus Rhythm

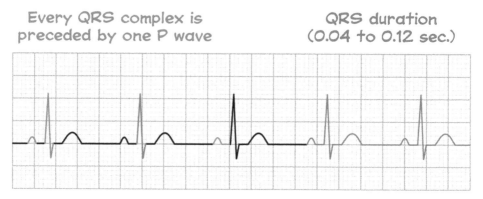

Every QRS complex is preceded by one P wave

QRS duration (0.04 to 0.12 sec.)

PR interval (0.12 to 0.20 sec.)

Rate and rhythm analysis	Normal values
Calculate the rate	60 to 100
Assess regularity	Regular
Check the P waves	Present, normal
Determine the QRS duration	0.04 to 0.12 seconds
Determine the PR interval	0.12 to 0.20 seconds
Determine the QT interval	Less than 0.46 seconds

Deviation from the normal values above may indicate the presence of sinus bradycardia, sinus tachycardia, or another arrhythmia.

It is important to note that sinus tachycardia often occurs as an appropriate response to stress. In addition, sinus bradycardia is commonly a normal finding in well conditioned athletes. There are, of course, pathologic causes to both of these conditions as well.

The Caliper

The caliper is a tool that can be used to measure relevant values on an ECG. It consists of two hinged legs with pointed tips. The tool has no intrinsic measuring ability of its own, but the width of the legs can be adjusted and measured against convenient portions of the ECG paper. The caliper method is also useful to assess the regularity of a rhythm.

Ensure the ECG is on a flat surface when using the caliper. To measure the ventricular rhythm, choose two consecutive R waves. Place one point of the caliper on the peak of the first R wave, then adjust the width of the caliper so that the other point of the caliper is on the subsequent R wave. This set distance is the RR interval. The caliper can now be pivoted against succeeding or preceding RR intervals to assess the regularity of the rhythm. A regular ventricular rhythm has RR intervals of the same length. If the RR intervals vary, then the ventricular rhythm is irregular.

The atrial rhythm is assessed by measuring the P-P intervals in a similar fashion. The distance between consecutive P waves should be consistent. Major variations in the P-P intervals indicate an irregular atrial rhythm.

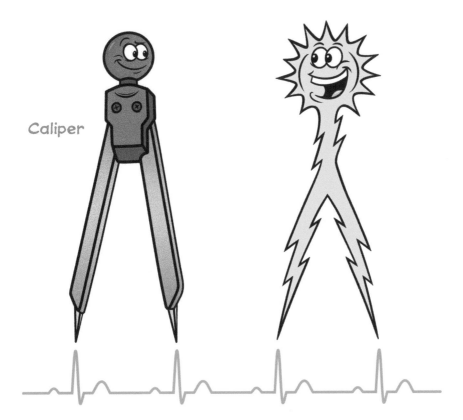

Caliper

Sparkson's Summary: Chapter 4

- The heart *rate* is described as the number of beats per minute. The heart *rhythm* refers to the pattern.

- The SA node generally maintains normal sinus rhythm at a rate between 60 and 100 beats per minute.

- The autonomic nervous system consists of the sympathetic nervous system (which stimulates the heart) and the parasympathetic nervous system (which inhibits the heart).

- Sinus bradycardia: sinus rhythm with a rate slower than 60 beats per minute.

- Sinus tachycardia: sinus rhythm with a rate faster than 100 beats per minute.

- Ectopic foci are potential pacemaker sites located outside of the SA node and function by overdrive suppression.

- The counting method for heart rates: find an R wave on a dark vertical line and use the next line to begin counting (300, 150, 100, 75, 60, 50). The position of the subsequent R wave determines the rate.

- P waves and QRS complexes normally correlate in a one to one fashion. AV dissociation occurs when the atria and ventricles beat independently.

- The caliper is a tool used to measure ECG values and assess the regularity of a rhythm.

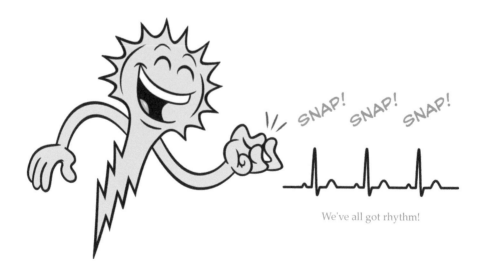

We've all got rhythm!

CHAPTER 5

AXIS

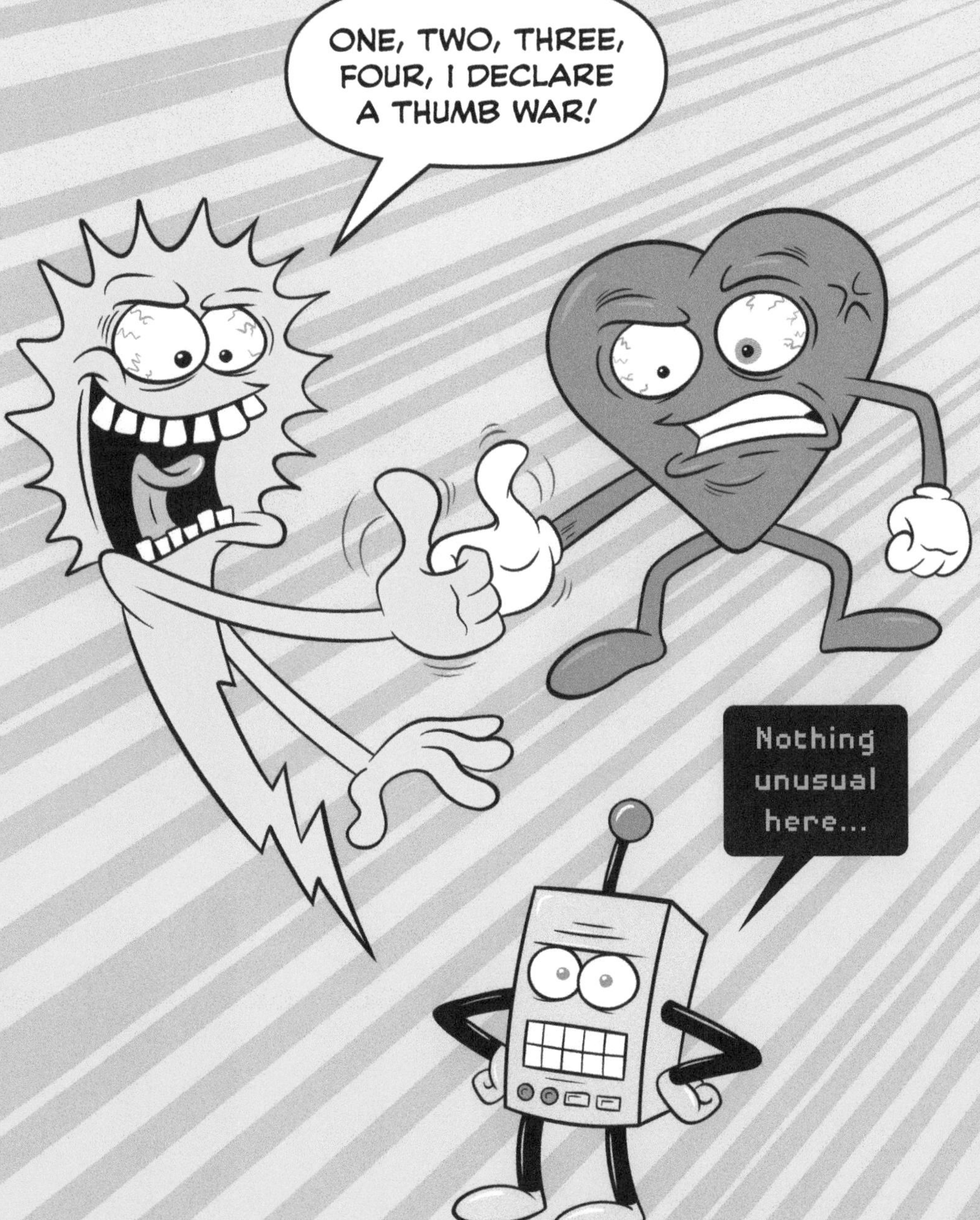

What's an Axis?

The *axis* of an ECG is the major direction of the overall electrical activity of the heart. This average movement of depolarization can be represented visually by a single arrow called a *vector*.

Depending on which direction the overall current is flowing, an axis may be normal, deviate leftward, deviate rightward, or demonstrate extreme deviation. Thus, we have four main labels to choose from when determining the axis of an ECG.

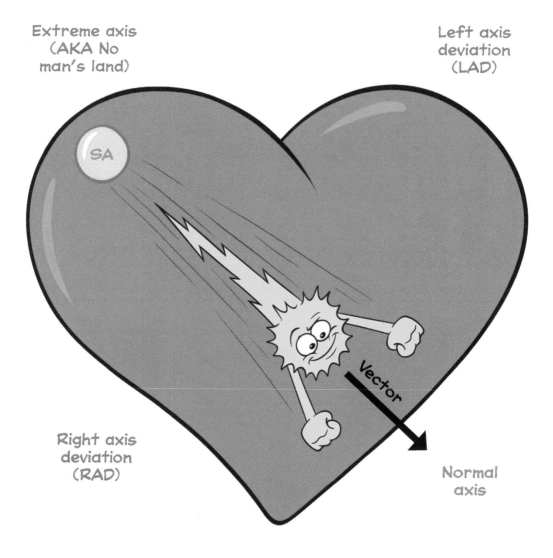

In a normal healthy heart, the average of all the depolarizations in the heart flows down and to the left from the SA node. The vector above points to a normal axis.

Mean QRS Vector

Smaller vectors can be used to demonstrate the direction of depolarization throughout the ventricles. The small vectors swing progressively to the left because the left ventricle is thicker than the right ventricle and dominates much of the electrical activity on the ECG. The average vector of all these small vectors is called the *mean QRS vector*.

The ECG's axis may change depending on certain pathologies affecting the conduction pathway. Axis deviation can provide insight into abnormalities of the conduction system, the origin of some arrhythmias, chamber enlargement, and myocardial infarction.

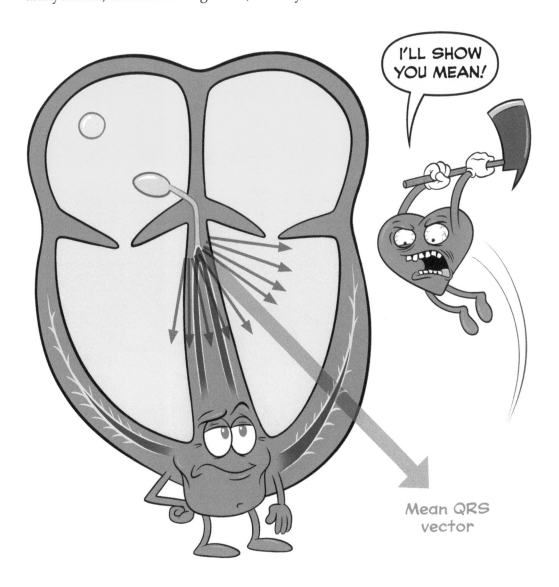

Mean QRS vector

The Hexaxial Reference System

The ECG's axis is illustrated as a circular schematic called the *hexaxial reference system*. The position of the mean QRS vector is described according to a number of degrees relative to a standardized circle. The vector's value on the schematic reveals whether it's pointing at a normal axis or at a deviated axis.

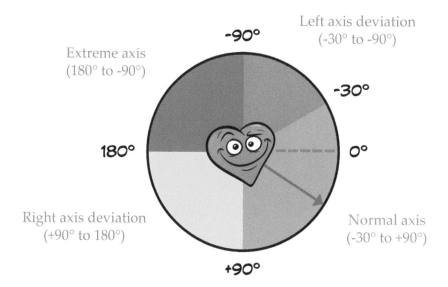

Theoretically speaking, this schematic represents the intersection of the six limb leads on the heart's frontal plane.

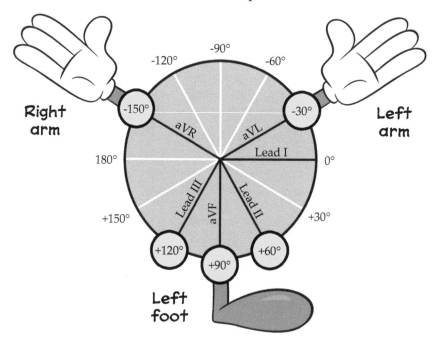

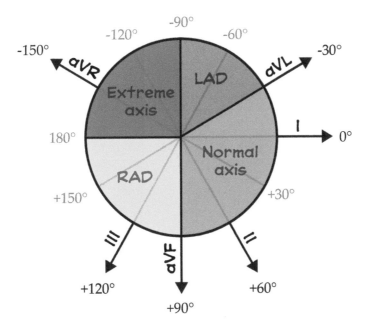

Before determining the axis of an ECG, we should review the classification of QRS complexes by morphology. The QRS complexes can be described according to the direction of their deflection relative to the isoelectric line (baseline).

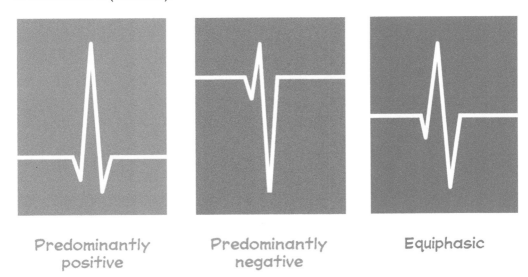

Predominantly positive | Predominantly negative | Equiphasic

Recall that positive deflections occur when depolarization flows towards a positive electrode, negative deflections occur when depolarization flows away from a positive electrode, and equiphasic deflections occur when depolarization flows perpendicular to a positive electrode. The absence of a deflection can also indicate that depolarization is traveling perpendicular to a positive electrode.

The Rule of Thumbs

The ECG's axis can be interpreted according to *the rule of thumbs.*
Let's assign a 'thumbs up' to a predominantly positive QRS deflection
and a 'thumbs down' to a predominantly negative QRS deflection. This
will make the technique of axis determination easier.

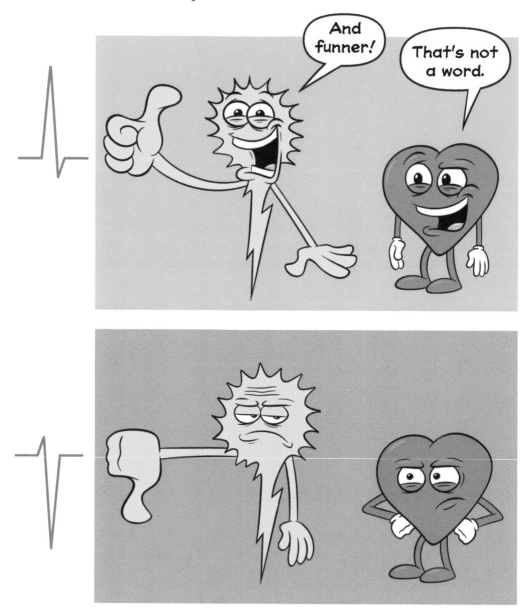

To assess the ECG's axis using the rule of thumbs, we only need to
focus on leads I, II, and aVF. For the most part we'll be comparing leads I
and aVF and referring to lead II as needed (PRN).

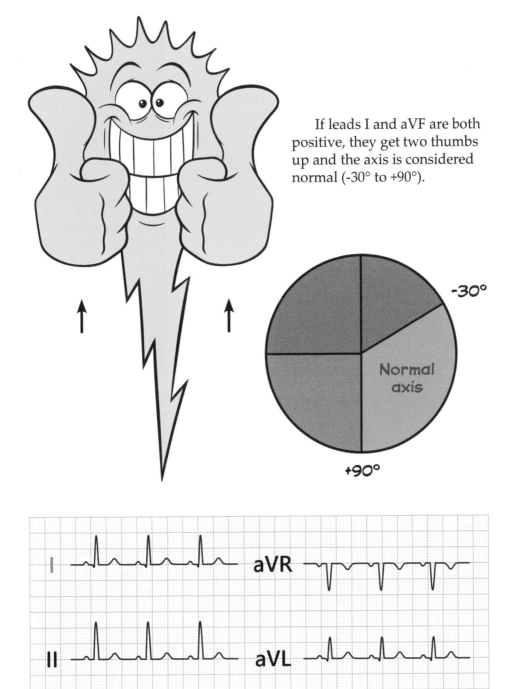

If leads I and aVF are both positive, they get two thumbs up and the axis is considered normal (-30° to +90°).

Normal axis (-30° to +90°)

85

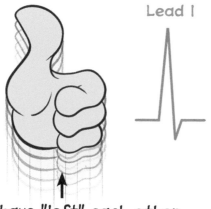

Lead I

Thumbs have "left" each other

Lead aVF

If lead I is positive and lead aVF is negative then they are given a thumb up and a thumb down, respectively. In this situation the thumbs have "left" each other which gives us an easy way to remember that there is possible left axis deviation.

However, in this case we should investigate further by looking at lead II. If lead II is positive, then the axis is considered normal (0° to -30°). If lead II is negative, then we can conclude that there is indeed left axis deviation (-30° to -90°).

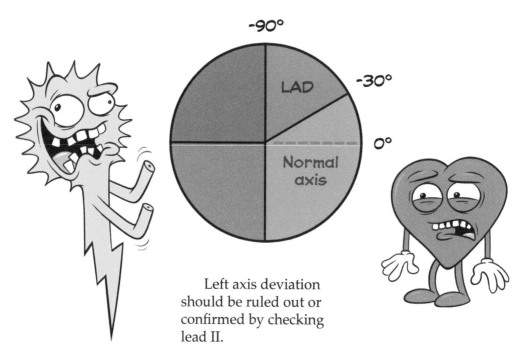

Left axis deviation should be ruled out or confirmed by checking lead II.

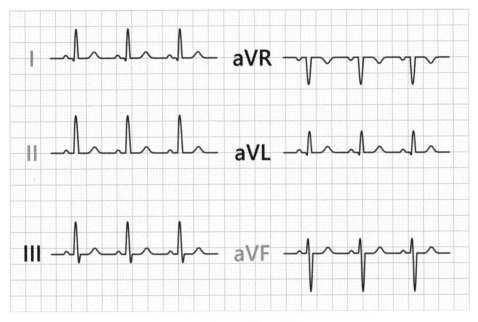

Normal axis (-30° to +90°)

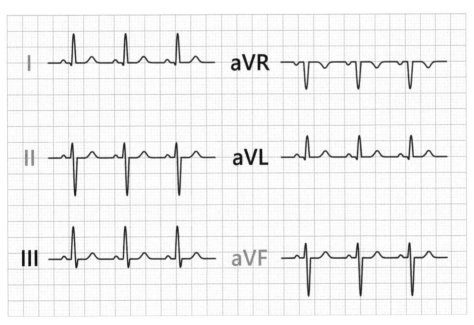

Left axis deviation (-30° to -90°)

Lead I

If lead I is negative and lead aVF is positive, then they are given a thumb down and a thumb up, respectively. Notice that the thumbs are headed "right" toward each other which gives us an easy to remember that there is right axis deviation. (+90° to 180°).

Lead aVF

180°

Thumbs are headed "right" toward each other

RAD

+90°

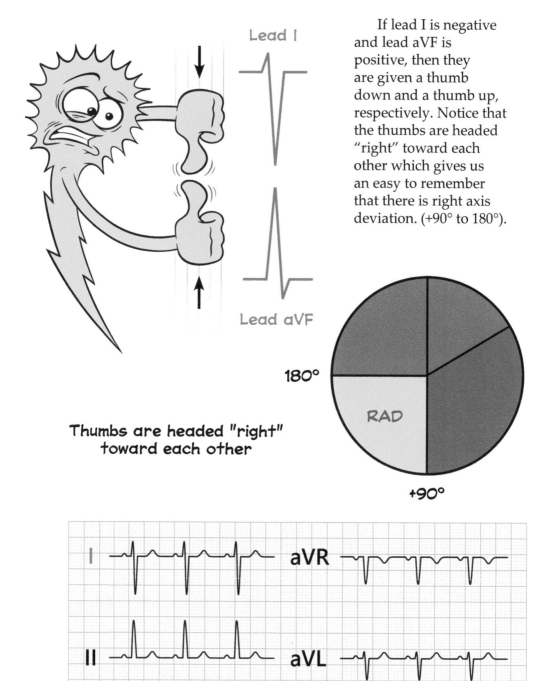

Right axis deviation (+90° to 180°)

If leads I and aVF are both negative, then they both get thumbs down and the axis is labeled as extreme (180° to -90°). We can easily remember this by noting that two thumbs down represents "extreme" disappointment.

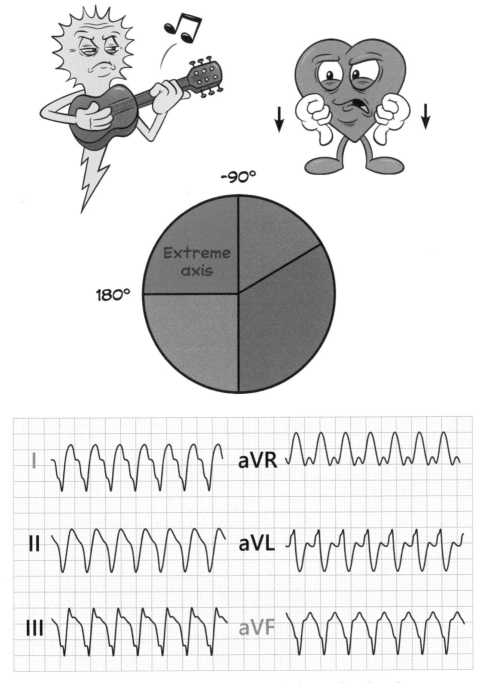

Extreme axis deviation (180° to -90°), example of ventricular tachycardia

Lead I		Lead aVF		Axis
Positive	∧	Positive	∧	Normal (-30° to +90°)
Positive	∧	Negative	∨	Possible LAD, thumbs "left" each other, check lead II Lead II positive: normal axis (0° to -30°) Lead II negative: left axis deviation (-30° to -90°)
Negative	∨	Positive	∧	RAD, thumbs headed "right" toward each other (+90° to 180°)
Negative	∨	Negative	∨	Extreme axis (180° to -90°)

Tip: when you're practicing this technique with your hands, keep your left thumb (lead I) above your right thumb (lead aVF). With a little practice you'll be able to quickly identify the axis without thumbing around, but this is a good way to get started.

You may have noticed that the rule of thumbs gives us a range of values for each axis category instead of a specific number in degrees. In clinical practice simply determining the axis category is usually sufficient, but situations may arise in which a more precise numerical estimate is desired. In these cases consider an alternative approach to axis interpretation is called the *equiphasic approach.*

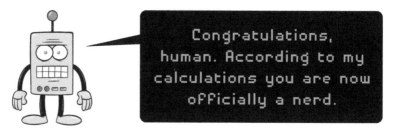

Congratulations, human. According to my calculations you are now officially a nerd.

The Equiphasic Approach

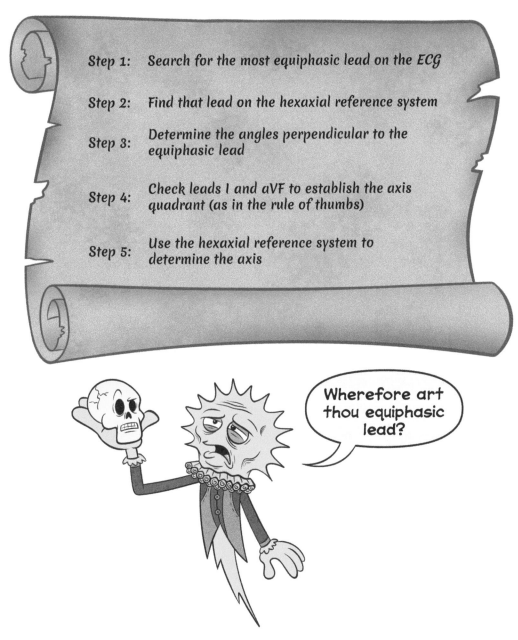

Step 1: Search for the most equiphasic lead on the ECG

Step 2: Find that lead on the hexaxial reference system

Step 3: Determine the angles perpendicular to the equiphasic lead

Step 4: Check leads I and aVF to establish the axis quadrant (as in the rule of thumbs)

Step 5: Use the hexaxial reference system to determine the axis

Wherefore art thou equiphasic lead?

The first step in the equiphasic approach is to search for the limb lead that contains the most equiphasic QRS complex. In other words, identify the limb lead that contains a QRS complex whose positive and negative deflections are approximately equal. In some instances the most equiphasic lead will appear flat, or isoelectric. Recall that an equiphasic QRS complex is recorded when depolarization flows perpendicular to a positive electrode.

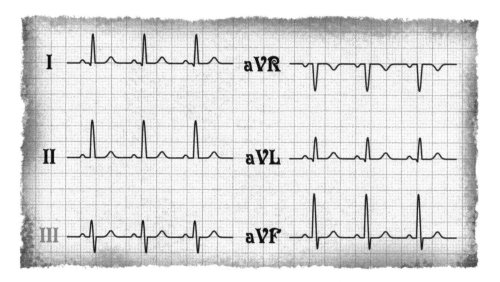

In the example above, lead III contains the most equiphasic QRS complex.

Identifying the most equiphasic QRS complex gives us an important piece of information about the orientation of the axis. We can now deduce that the mean QRS vector is pointing perpendicular (at a 90° angle) to the most equiphasic lead.

To properly visualize this concept, we'll need to look back at our handy hexaxial reference system. Let's continue to use lead III as the most equiphasic lead in our example.

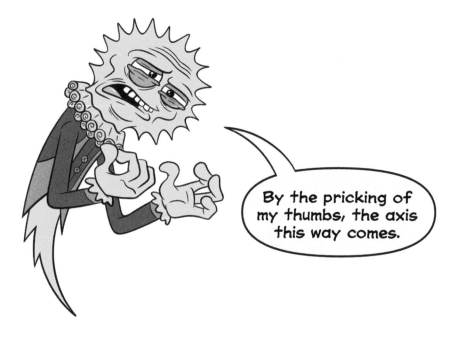

By the pricking of my thumbs, the axis this way comes.

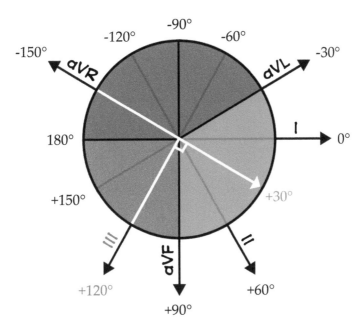

Lead III has a standard orientation of 120°. An equiphasic QRS complex at lead III puts the possible axis at -150° or +30°. At this point we can use the rule of thumbs to decide in which quadrant the axis lies. In our example leads I and aVF were both positive. Therefore, the ECG gets two thumbs up for a normal axis, and the precise angle of orientation is determined to be +30°.

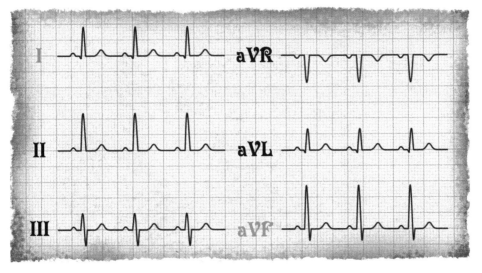

The axis is oriented perpendicularly to the most equiphasic limb lead

Determine the axis of the ECG below using the equiphasic approach:

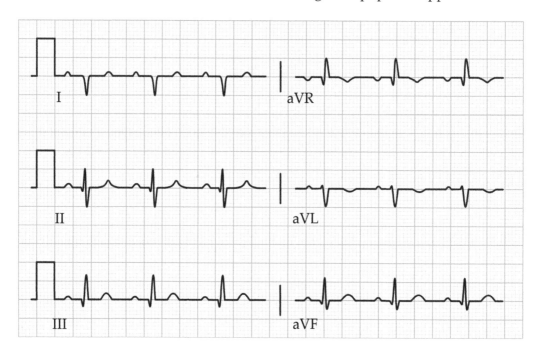

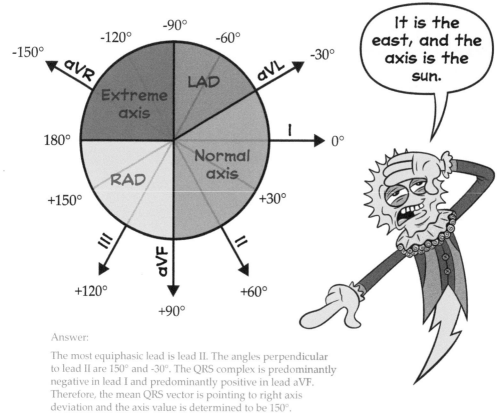

It is the east, and the axis is the sun.

Answer:

The most equiphasic lead is lead II. The angles perpendicular to lead II are 150° and -30°. The QRS complex is predominantly negative in lead I and predominantly positive in lead aVF. Therefore, the mean QRS vector is pointing to right axis deviation and the axis value is determined to be 150°.

Causes of Axis Deviation

Left axis deviation

- Left anterior fascicular block
- Left bundle branch block (LBBB)
- Inferior myocardial infarction
- Artificial cardiac pacing
- Wolff-Parkinson-White syndrome
- Ostium primum defect (ASD)
- Left ventricular hypertrophy (controversial)

Right axis deviation

- Left posterior fascicular block
- Lateral myocardial infarction
- Chronic obstructive pulmonary disease (COPD)
- Pulmonary embolus (PE)
- Right ventricular hypertrophy
- Normal finding in children or tall thin adults
- Wolff-Parkinson-White syndrome
- Dextrocardia

Extreme axis

- Ventricular rhythms (e.g. ventricular tachycardia)
- Severe right ventricular hypertrophy
- Hyperkalemia
- Limb lead reversal
- Artificial cardiac pacing
- Emphysema

Note: on occasion you may encounter an ECG in which all six limb leads appear equiphasic. In this case the axis is said to be *indeterminate*.

Effect of Positional Anomalies on Axis

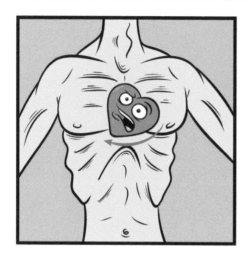

Vertical heart: right axis deviation may be seen in tall, slender individuals due to clockwise rotation of the heart towards the right side.

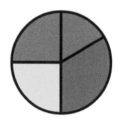

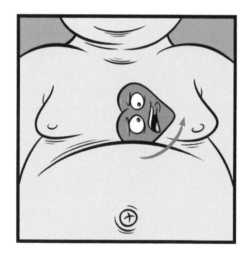

Horizontal heart: left axis deviation may be seen in morbidly obese individuals due to displacement of the heart by an elevated diaphragm in the supine position.

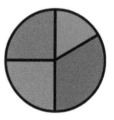

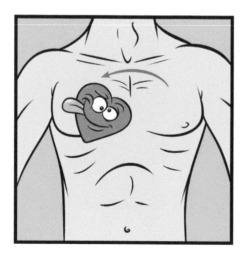

Dextrocardia: is a condition in which the apex of the heart is positioned toward the right side of the chest. The locations of the chambers are variable and there is right axis deviation.

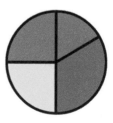

Dextrocardia

Dextrocardia is a positional anomaly of the heart with several characteristic ECG features:

- Inversion of all complexes in lead I (global negativity)

- Positive complexes in lead aVR

- Right axis deviation

- Reverse or absent R wave progression in the precordial leads

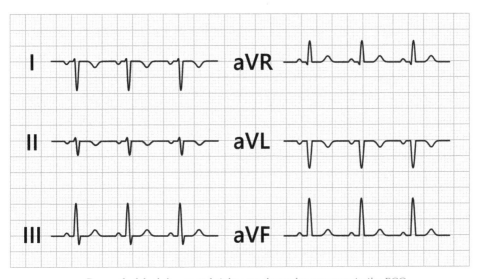

Reversal of the left arm and right arm electrodes causes a similar ECG pattern in the limb leads, but the precordial leads are not affected

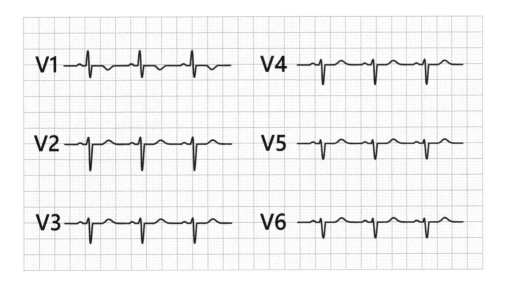

Sparkson's Summary: Chapter 5

- The axis is the major direction of the heart's electrical activity and may deviate from normal in the setting of cardiovascular disease.

- The hexaxial reference system is a visual representation of the axis utilizing a vector arrow pointed at a numerical value (in degrees).

- Normal axis: -30° to +90° (both thumbs up).

- Left axis deviation: -30° to -90° (have "left" each other).

- Right axis deviation: +90° to 180° (are headed "right" at each other).

- Extreme axis: 180° to -90° (both thumbs down).

- The equiphasic approach provides a more precise numerical estimate of the axis, but is less commonly used in clinical practice.

- There are numerous causes of axis deviation which vary from benign to life-threatening.

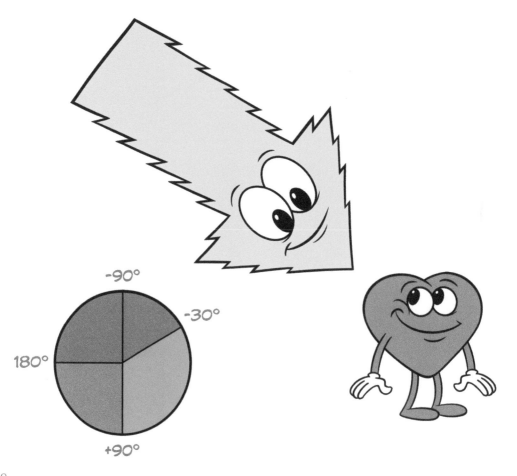

CHAPTER 6

HYPERTROPHY AND ENLARGEMENT

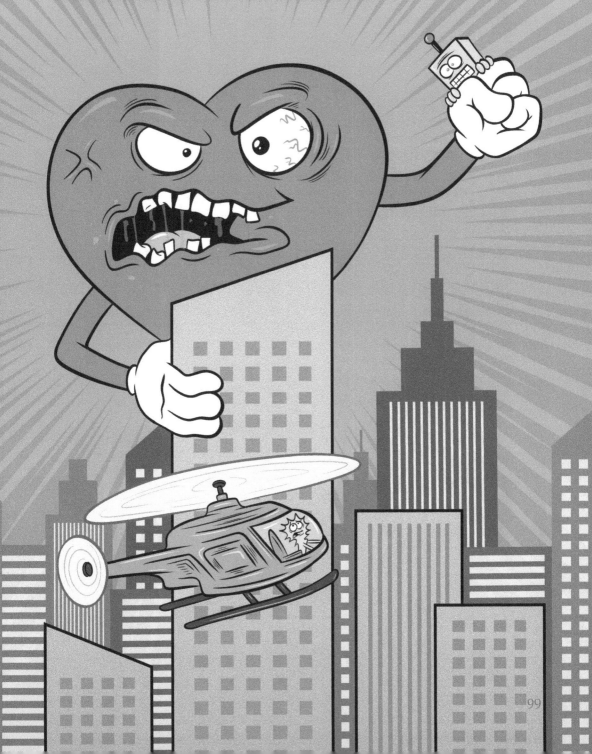

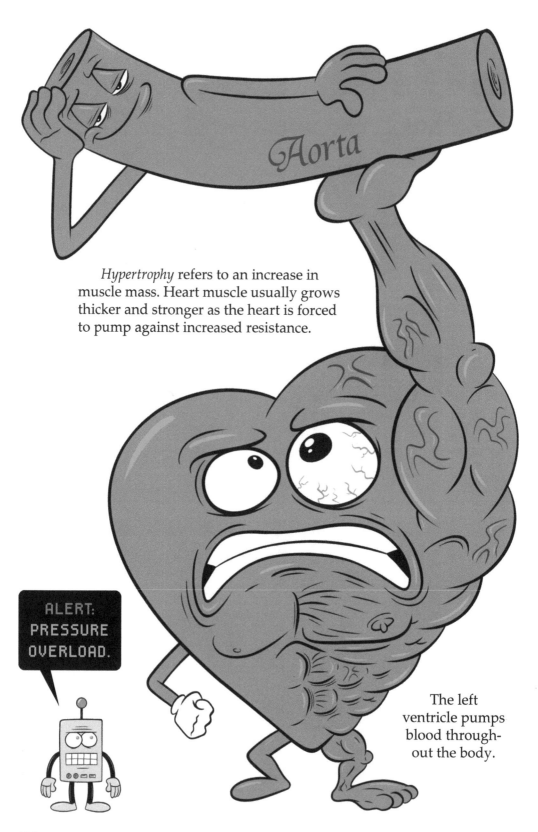

Hypertrophy refers to an increase in muscle mass. Heart muscle usually grows thicker and stronger as the heart is forced to pump against increased resistance.

ALERT: PRESSURE OVERLOAD.

The left ventricle pumps blood throughout the body.

Enlargement refers to dilation of a particular chamber of the heart. The space inside the chamber increases to accommodate an increased amount of blood.

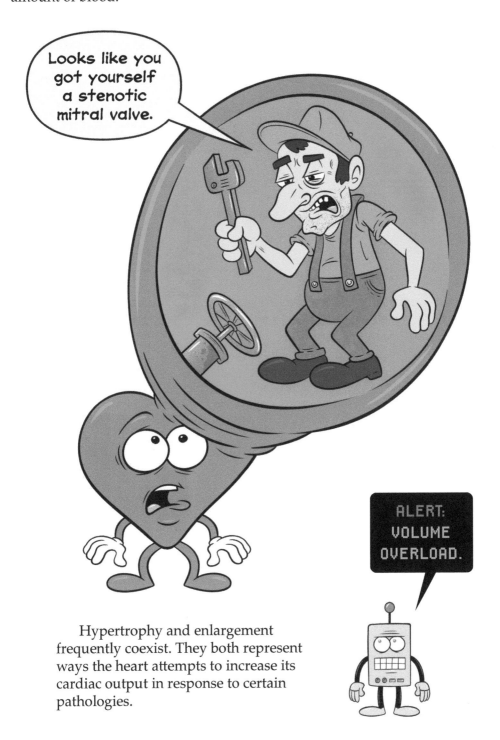

Hypertrophy and enlargement frequently coexist. They both represent ways the heart attempts to increase its cardiac output in response to certain pathologies.

If hypertrophy or enlargement is present, then the electric impulse has a longer distance to travel through the heart. This is reflected in a wave by an increase in its duration.

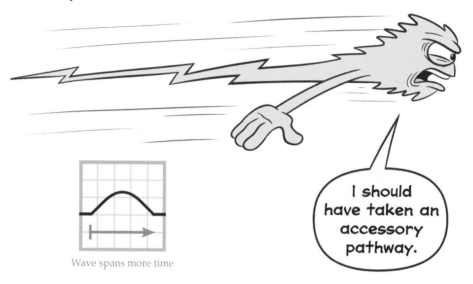

I should have taken an accessory pathway.

Wave spans more time

An increase in voltage may be seen with greater amounts of cardiac tissue for the electric impulse to travel through. This manifests in a wave by an increase in its amplitude.

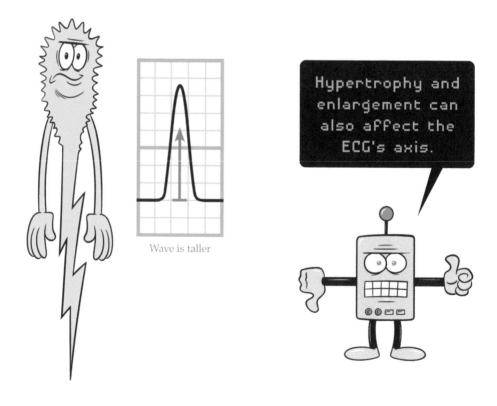

Wave is taller

Hypertrophy and enlargement can also affect the ECG's axis.

The P wave and Atrial Enlargement

The P wave represents the depolarization and simultaneous contraction of both atria. It is therefore our best source for evidence of atrial enlargement.

We can focus our attention on leads II and V1. Limb lead II provides a good monophasic deflection of the P wave because it is oriented nearly parallel to the flow of electricity through the atria.

Lead V1 may be even more useful because the chest electrode that records V1 is positioned directly over the atria. Furthermore, lead V1 usually produces a biphasic P wave because it is oriented perpendicular to the normal flow of electricity.

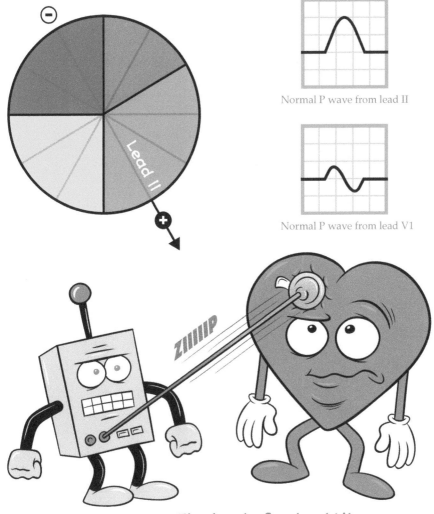

Normal P wave from lead II

Normal P wave from lead V1

Electrode for lead V1

The P wave can be separated into a right atrial component and a left atrial component. Each component represents right and left atrial depolarization, respectively, and they will morph depending on whether atrial enlargement is present. The right and left atrial components are also known as the initial and terminal components, respectively.

Normal P wave from lead II

Right atrial component (initial component)   **Left atrial component (terminal component)**

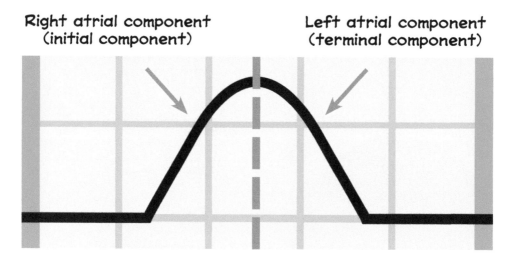

Normal P wave from lead VI

Right atrial component (initial component)   **Left atrial component (terminal component)**

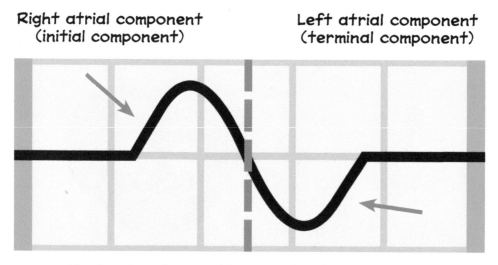

The duration of a normal P wave is less than 0.12 seconds. The amplitude of a normal P wave, whether positive or negative, is less than 2.5 mm in the limb leads, and less than 1.5 mm in the precordial leads. Consider atrial enlargement when the P wave deviates from these parameters.

Right Atrial Enlargement

The primary deformity to the P wave in right atrial enlargement (RAE) is an increase in amplitude. RAE can be diagnosed by identifying P waves with an amplitude greater than 2.5 mm in the inferior leads (II, III, and aVF). In lead V1, RAE causes the right atrial component of the P wave to rise higher than 1.5 mm.

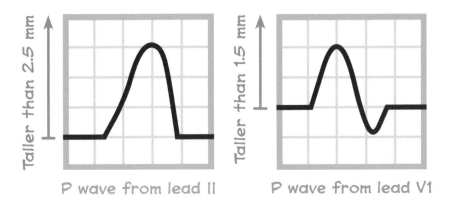

P wave from lead II — P wave from lead V1

RAE is also known as *P pulmonale* because it can be caused by severe lung disease. The causes of RAE include pulmonary hypertension, chronic lung disease, tricuspid stenosis, and congenital heart disease (e.g. pulmonary stenosis and tetralogy of Fallot).

The primary cause of **RAE** is pulmonary hypertension.

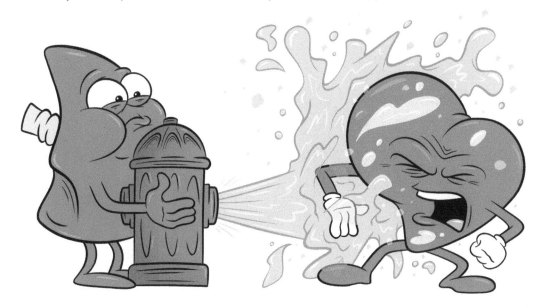

Left Atrial Enlargement

Left atrial enlargement (LAE) is characterized by an increase in the P wave's duration, giving the wave a widened appearance. This is commonly seen in lead II when the P wave spans 0.12 seconds or greater.

In lead V1, the terminal component of the P wave will span 0.04 seconds or greater and drop at least 1 mm below the isoelectric line.

LAE is also known as *P mitrale* because the condition is classically seen with mitral stenosis. The P wave in lead II may develop a notched appearance, consisting of a distinct second peak often described as appearing "m-like" in shape.

LAE is also associated with conditions that cause left ventricular hypertrophy (e.g. systemic hypertension, aortic stenosis, mitral valve incompetence, and hypertrophic cardiomyopathy).

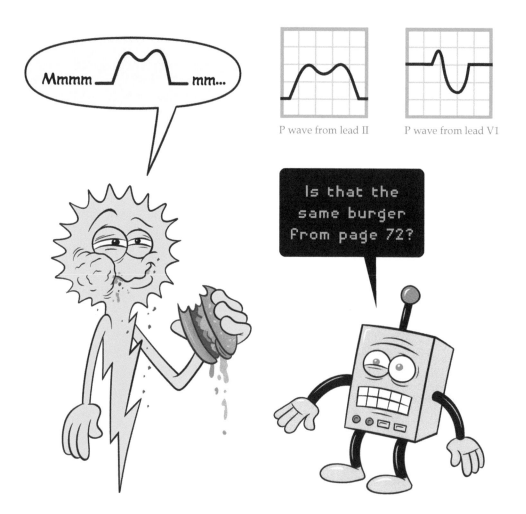

P wave from lead II   P wave from lead V1

R Wave Progression

The QRS complex represents ventricular depolarization and the initiation of ventricular contraction. Cardiac conduction begins on the right side of the heart and flows down and to the left. Relative to the chest leads, the electrical impulse therefore travels from V1 to V6.

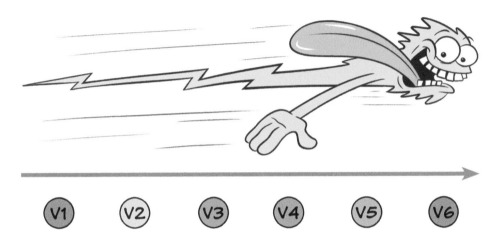

Normal progression of the QRS complex from V1 to V6

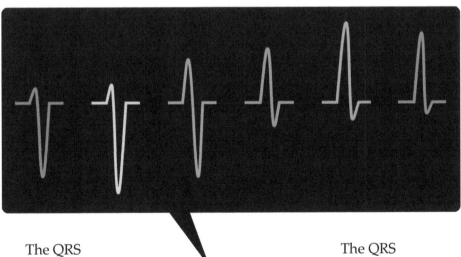

The QRS complex begins with a predominantly negative deflection in V1 and V2 because depolarization is traveling away from the positive electrodes.

The QRS complex ends with a predominantly positive deflection in V5 and V6 because depolarization is traveling toward the positive electrodes.

Right Ventricular Hypertrophy

In right ventricular hypertrophy (RVH), the right ventricle is very thick. Thus, there is much more electricity flowing in its direction, producing a large R wave in lead V1. There will also be a large S wave in lead V5 or V6.

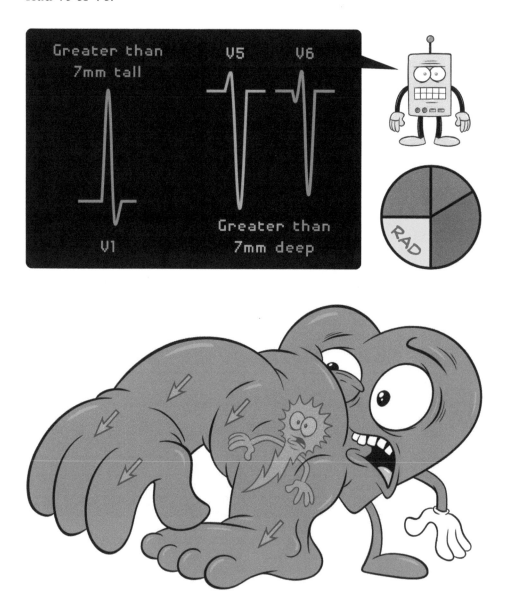

RVH causes right axis deviation (RAD) of +110° or more because the increase in muscle mass adds more vectors to the right side. The most common causes of RVH are pulmonary hypertension, mitral stenosis, pulmonary embolism, and congenital heart disease.

Left Ventricular Hypertrophy

In left ventricular hypertrophy (LVH) the left side of the heart wall is very thick, which exaggerates the deflection of the QRS complex in the chest leads.

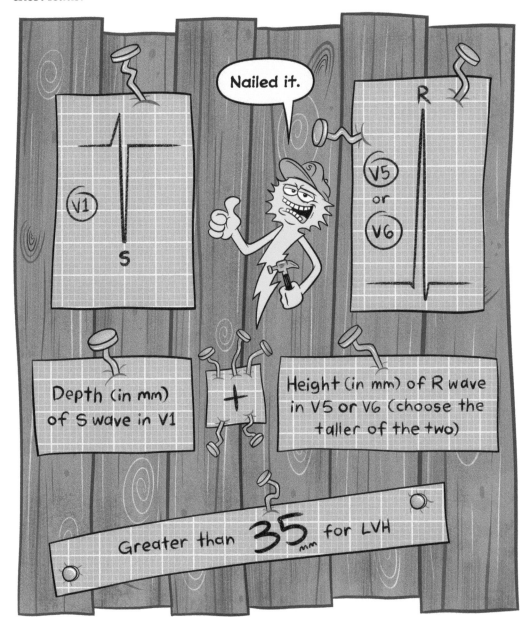

If the sum of the depth of the S wave in V1 and the height of the R wave in V5 or V6 is greater than 35 mm, then there is evidence of LVH. Now turn to page 35 and look at the bottom right corner to reinforce this concept.

There are many different sets of criteria that have been proposed for the diagnosis of LVH. The formula on the previous page is one example of voltage criteria (and the most popular).

It is called voltage criteria because the diagnostic parameters depend on the amplitude of the wave. Other examples of voltage criteria include:

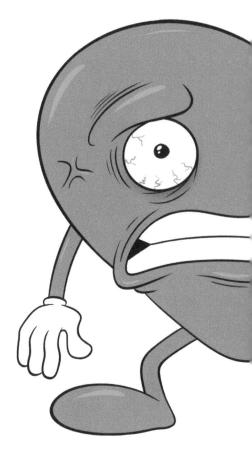

Limb leads

- R wave in lead I + S wave in lead III > 25 mm
- R wave in aVL > 11 mm
- R wave in aVF > 20 mm

Precordial leads

- R wave in V5 > 26 mm
- R wave in V6 > 18 mm
- R wave in V5 > V6

The sensitivity and specificity of these criteria vary and none of them are perfect. The more criteria that are positive for the same ECG, the more likely that LVH is present.

False positives are frequently seen in young or thin individuals, whose voltage may exceed conventional parameters.

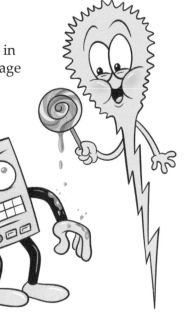

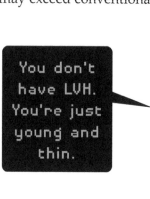

You don't have LVH. You're just young and thin.

The most common cause of LVH is hypertension. Other causes include aortic stenosis, aortic regurgitation (AKA aortic insufficiency), mitral regurgitation (AKA mitral insufficiency), coarctation of the aorta, and hypertrophic cardiomyopathy.

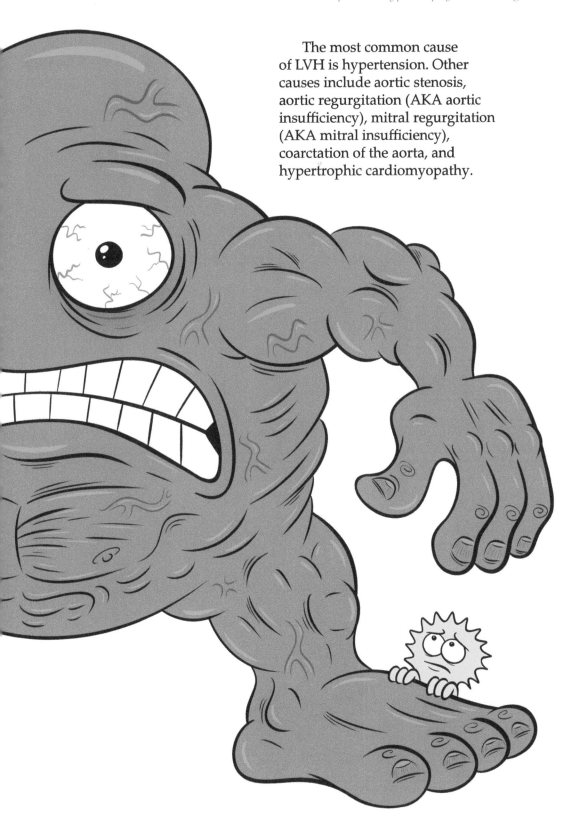

Repolarization Abnormalities

Hypertrophy of a ventricle may result in the appearance of repolarization abnormalities on the ECG. These ECG changes generally manifest as ST depression and asymmetric T wave inversion. These repolarization abnormalities are often referred to as the ventricular "strain" pattern.

Right ventricular repolarization abnormalities will be most evident in leads V1 and V2. Left ventricular repolarization abnormalities will be most evident in leads I, aVL, V5, and V6.

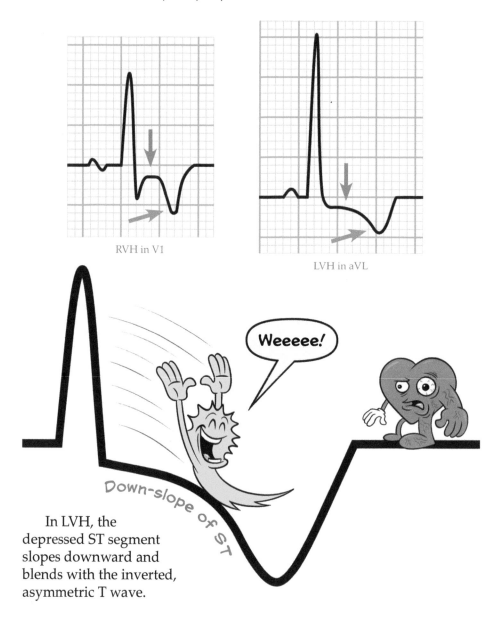

RVH in V1

LVH in aVL

Down-slope of ST

Weeeee!

In LVH, the depressed ST segment slopes downward and blends with the inverted, asymmetric T wave.

Echocardiography

Although the ECG is a useful tool in the analysis of cardiac chamber abnormalities, it is not always reliable. In many cases the test will have low diagnostic sensitivity or result in ECG findings that are nonspecific.

Echocardiography is a more accurate method to investigate hypertrophy and enlargement. An echocardiogram (echo) is a test that utilizes ultrasound to visualize the heart. It provides information about the size and shape of the cardiac chambers and surrounding structures, function and morphology of the valves, systolic and diastolic function, and ejection fraction.

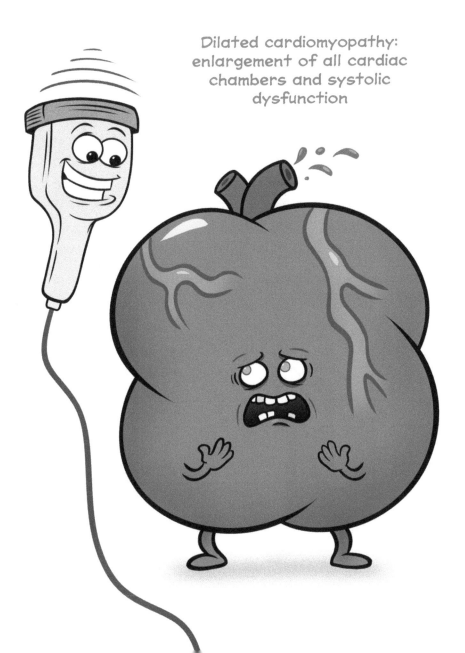

Dilated cardiomyopathy: enlargement of all cardiac chambers and systolic dysfunction

Sparkson's Summary: Chapter 6

- Hypertrophy: refers to an increase in muscle mass.

- Enlargement: refers to cardiac chamber dilation.

- An abnormally wide ECG wave reflects a prolongation in the depolarization time.

- Right atrial enlargement

  - Lead II: P wave taller than 2.5 mm

  - Lead V1: P wave taller than 1.5 mm

- Left atrial enlargement

  - Lead II: P wave widening of 0.12 seconds or greater (m-like)

  - Lead V1: P wave terminal component widening of 0.04 seconds or greater and depression of at least 1 mm below baseline

- Right ventricular hypertrophy: R wave in V1 greater than 7 mm tall and S wave in lead V5 or V6 greater than 7 mm deep.

- Left ventricular hypertrophy: sum of S wave depth in V1 and R wave height in V5 or V6 greater than 35 mm (Sokolow-Lyon criteria).

- Hypertrophy of a ventricle may result in ECG changes such as axis deviation and repolarization abnormalities.

- Echocardiogram: a diagnostic tool to assess the structures and function of the heart.

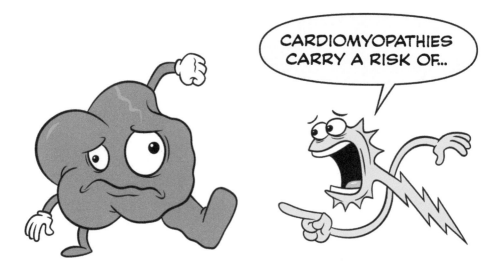

CARDIOMYOPATHIES CARRY A RISK OF...

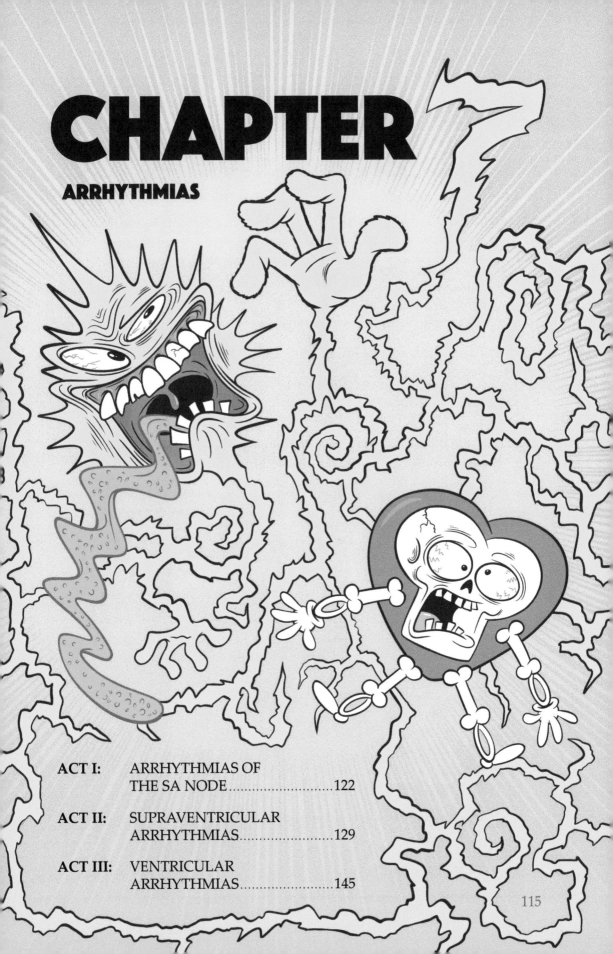

CHAPTER 7

ARRHYTHMIAS

115

Arrhythmias

An arrhythmia, or dysrhythmia, is any rhythm that deviates from normal sinus rhythm. Chapter 4 (Rate and Rhythm) laid the foundation for the concepts you'll need to know to identify arrhythmias on an ECG.

Some arrhythmias are relatively harmless
(e.g. premature atrial contraction)

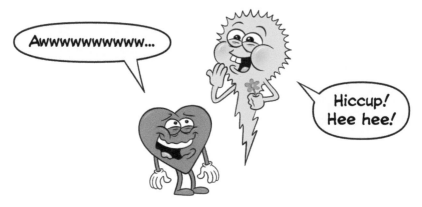

Other arrhythmias are dangerous and can cause sudden cardiac death
(e.g. ventricular fibrillation)

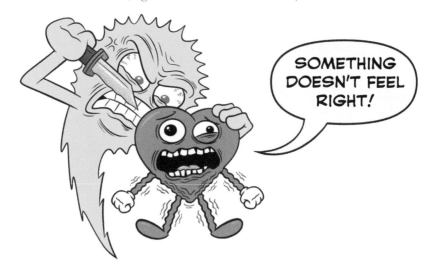

An arrhythmia that is caused by a delay or interruption of cardiac conduction is termed a heart block. These types of arrhythmias will be discussed in greater detail in chapter 8.

An arrhythmia that originates above the level of the bundle of His is called a supraventricular arrhythmia. Furthermore, if the rate is greater than 100 beats per minute, then the arrhythmia is called a supraventricular tachycardia (SVT).

The heart's normal rhythm can be disturbed by a variety of factors.

Structual changes
- Enlargement and hypertrophy
- Valvular disease
- Congenital disorders

Hypoxia
- Chronic obstructive pulmonary disease (COPD)
- Pulmonary embolism (PE)
- Obstructive sleep apnea (OSA)

Autonomic nervous system
- Hyperthyroidism or hypothyroidism
- Bradycardia
- Nervousness

Drugs
- Many drugs and medications
- Alcohol
- Caffeine

Electrolyte abnormalities
- Imbalances of potassium
- Imbalances of calcium
- Imbalances of magnesium

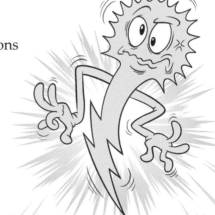

Ambulatory ECG Monitoring

The standard 12-lead ECG captures the heart's electrical activity over a limited period of time. Ambulatory ECG monitoring is used to capture extended electrocardiographic data. This technique is useful for any arrhythmic activity that might be of brief duration and not easily detectable with a standard ECG.

Clinically, ambulatory ECG monitoring is indicated in cases of unexplained syncope or unexplained recurrent palpitations.

A Holter monitor is a portable ECG device that can store a complete record of the heart's rhythm over a 24 to 48 hour period. Similar to standard electrocardiography, the unit usually employs two or three electrodes placed on the chest to record its leads.

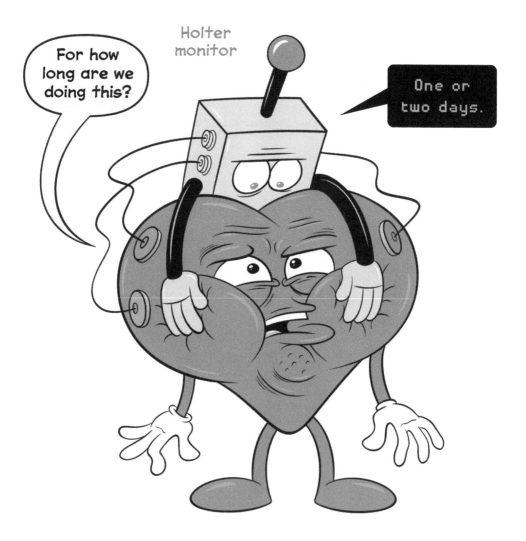

An event monitor is a device used when symptoms suspicious for an arrhythmia occur infrequently. It is typically worn for several weeks and can be activated by the patient when symptoms arise.

Surgically implanted event recorders are also available which can record the heart's electrical activity over a span of months to years.

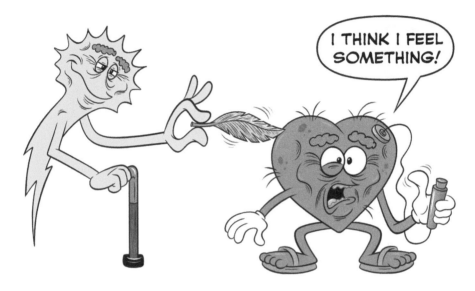

The technology of ambulatory ECG monitoring continues to evolve with the emergence of smartphones and apps. Wireless ambulatory ECGs are one such example. These devices utilize technologies such as Bluetooth to transmit data to a patient's smartphone. The report may then be shared with a clinician through a secure Internet connection.

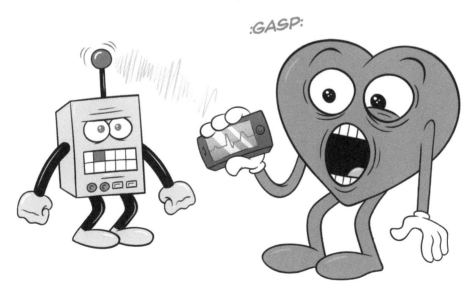

Reentry

In a healthy heart, an electric impulse traveling down muscle tissue will eventually meet a fork in the road, at which point the impulse will split and conduct along both branches. If the two branches are connected together by a common branch, the impulses will split again. The impulses traveling toward each other in the common branch cancel each other out, while the other branching impulses continue to propagate down through the myocardium.

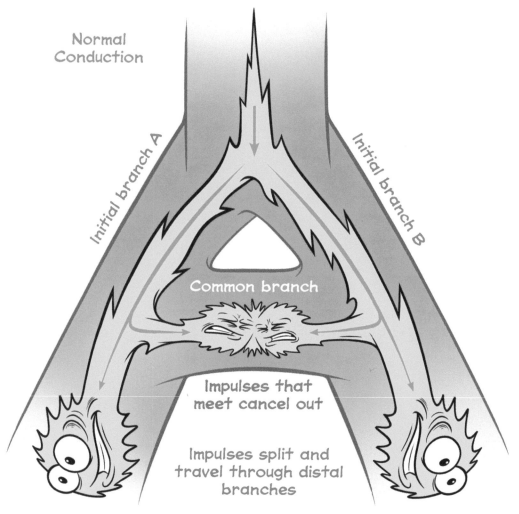

Normal Conduction

Initial branch A

Initial branch B

Common branch

Impulses that meet cancel out

Impulses split and travel through distal branches

Reentry represents an abnormality in the transmission of electric impulses through the heart. The term "reentry" refers to an electrophysiologic mechanism in which an electric impulse gets caught in a loop. It is a common cause of many clinically important arrhythmias. Reentry can occur in one small area of the heart (such as the AV node), affect an entire chamber, or involve both the atrium and the ventricle.

Reentry can occur due to *anatomic* or *functional* disturbances in the myocardium. Examples of anatomic abnormalities include scarring from infarcted tissue and congenital accessory pathways. Functional disturbances arise due to electrophysiological variation within the myocardium. Functional disturbances can occur as a consequence of input from the ANS or from the intrinsic properties of cardiomyocytes (e.g. cardiac cells causing premature depolarization).

In the process of reentry, one of the initial branches transmits the electric impulse more slowly than the other. The region of slowed conduction is said to have a "unidirectional block" because it only affects the velocity of an electric impulse traveling antegrade (forward) through the pathway.

As the impulse traveling down the unaffected branch enters the common branch, it finds that it is able to travel back to the starting point by entering the blocked pathway in a retrograde fashion. This process can create a revolving circuit that overdrives the SA node.

Whether or not the counter-clockwise reentry loop is sustained depends on the excitability of the cardiac tissue at the starting point. If the tissue is still in a refractory period, then the loop would be terminated.

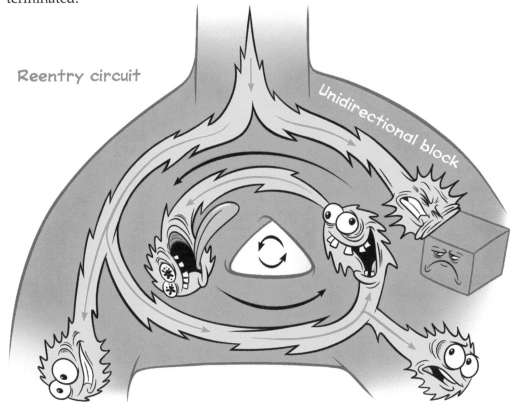

Reentry circuit

Unidirectional block

Respiratory Sinus Arrhythmia

The ECG will often demonstrate minor variations in the distance between successive P waves. This is a normal physiologic mechanism in which the heart rate increases gradually during inspiration and decreases with expiration.

The variation is attributed to varying levels of stimulation and inhibition of the SA node from the autonomic nervous system (ANS). The *vagus nerve* is a component of the ANS that's responsible for slowing the heart rate. Inspiration stretches the lung tissue and causes a reflex inhibition of vagal tone, which increases the heart rate. During expiration vagal tone is no longer inhibited, and the heart rate slows back down.

Minor variations in the P to P intervals during respiration is a normal phenomenon

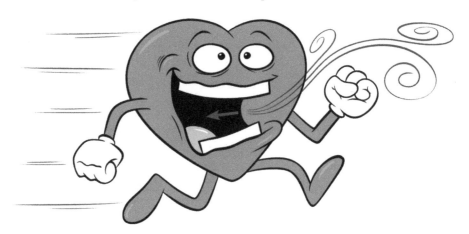

Inspiration accelerates the heart rate

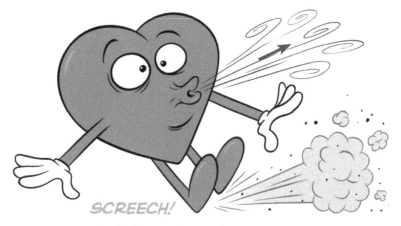

SCREECH!

Exhalation slows the heart rate

Sinus Bradycardia

Sinus bradycardia is present when the SA node paces the heart at a rate slower than 60 beats per minute. It's not usually considered clinically significant unless the rate drops below 50 beats per minute. Extremely slow heart rates may cause symptoms such as lightheadedness, syncope, or worsening angina pectoris.

Sinus bradycardia is frequently encountered as a normal finding in healthy athletes at rest. In these individuals vagal tone increases with endurance training.

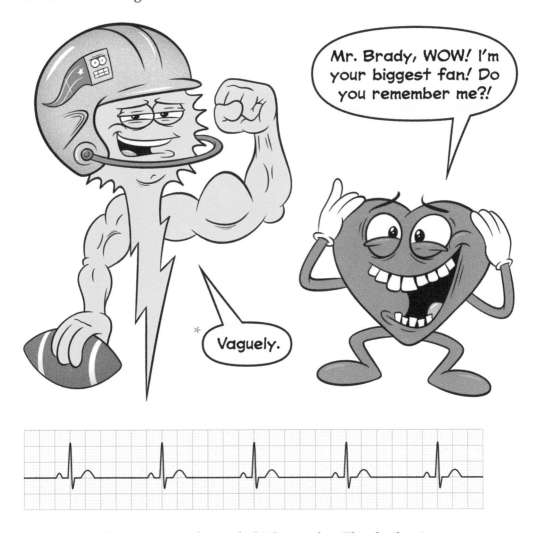

A normal P wave precedes each QRS complex. The rhythm is regular, as noted by the consistent R to R intervals.

* Brady makes a reference to the vagus nerve.

Sinus Tachycardia

If the SA node fires at a rate greater than 100 times per minute, it is called sinus tachycardia. While the frequency of impulses increases, the rhythm remains regular.

Sinus tachycardia is most commonly induced by exercise due to increased sympathetic stimulation of the SA node. Other causes include anxiety, the consumption of drugs or alcohol, and a variety of disease states (e.g. fever, hypotension, hypoxia, anemia, and pheochromocytoma, among others).

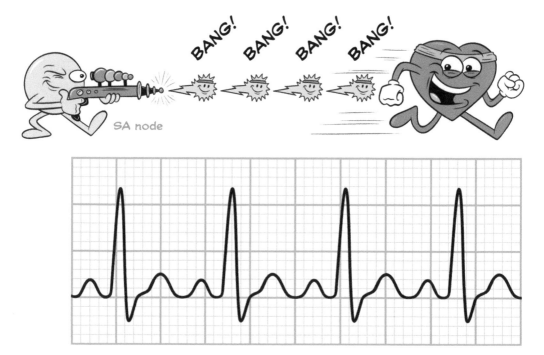

With very fast heart rates, the P wave may merge with the preceding T wave, producing a "camel hump" appearance.

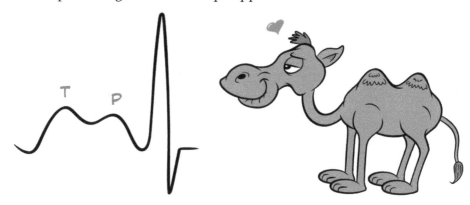

Sinus Pause and Arrest

Sinus pause is a temporary failure of depolarization from the SA node.

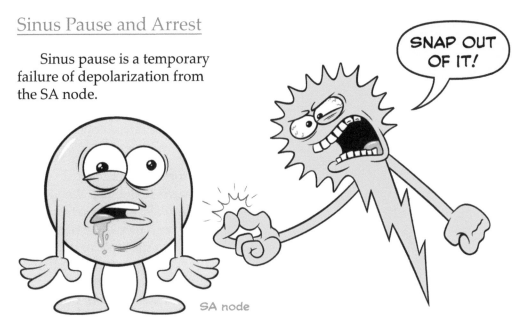

SA node

If this inactivity is prolonged and marked by the absence of P waves, then the condition is called sinus arrest. Overdrive suppression is usually triggered from an ectopic focus, and the rescue beat is called an *escape beat*.

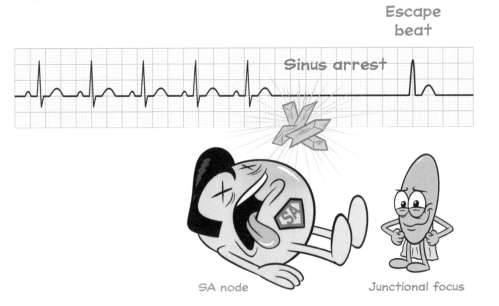

Escape beat

Sinus arrest

SA node

Junctional focus

In the example above of sinus arrest, a junctional focus has stepped in to provide pacing. We can infer that the escape beat did not originate from the atria because there is no P wave accompanying the rescue. However, a junctional escape beat can sometimes produce an inverted P' wave before or after the QRS complex known as a *retrograde P wave*.

Sinoatrial Exit Block

If the SA node is able to generate an impulse, but fails to transmit the impulse out and into the atria, then the condition is referred to as sinoatrial exit block. This arrhythmia manifests on the ECG as a transient flatline similar to sinus pause or sinus arrest. Sinoatrial exit block may be caused by impaired automaticity of the SA node, impaired conduction to the surrounding tissue, or both.

Sinoatrial exit block can be distinguished from transient sinus arrest by analyzing the P to P intervals. In sinoatrial exit block the SA node discharges electric impulses at regular intervals, but one or more cycles don't appear on the ECG. When sinoatrial exit block resolves, depolarization of the atria resumes on the ECG as a multiple of the normal P to P interval (e.g. there will be *exactly* one, two, or more missed P waves). Sinus pause and transient sinus arrest do not demonstrate such a pattern and the SA node resumes pacing at any random point on the ECG tracing.

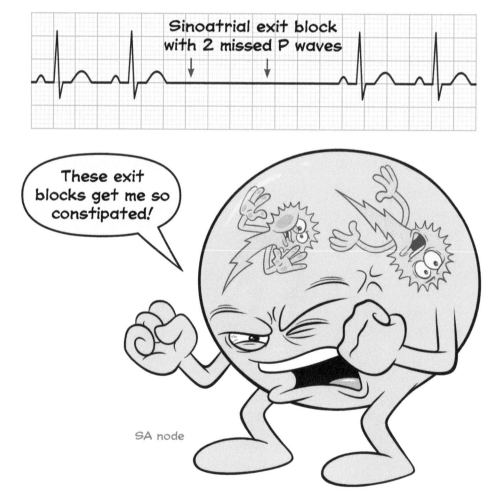

Sick Sinus Syndrome

Sick sinus syndrome (SSS) refers to a spectrum of arrhythmias associated with a dysfunctional SA node. The conditions encompassed by SSS include: inappropriate sinus bradycardia, sinus pause or arrest, sinoatrial exit block, and alternating bradycardia with atrial *tachyarrhythmias. *Bradycardia-tachycardia syndrome* describes the variant of SSS involving alternating bradycardia with atrial tachyarrhythmias.

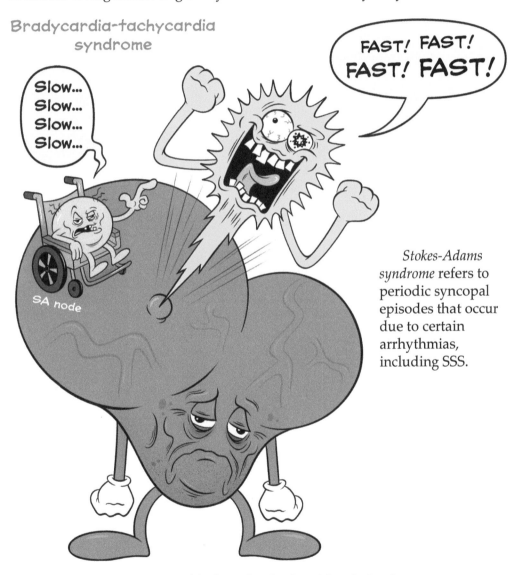

Bradycardia-tachycardia syndrome

Slow... Slow... Slow... Slow...

FAST! FAST! FAST! FAST!

SA node

Stokes-Adams syndrome refers to periodic syncopal episodes that occur due to certain arrhythmias, including SSS.

SSS is most common in elderly individuals with existing heart disease. Treatment involves the removal of precipitating factors (e.g. non-essential drugs) or artificial pacemaker insertion.

* Fast and abnormal rhythms.

Premature Atrial Complexes (PACs)

A premature atrial complex is a premature beat generated from an ectopic focus within the atria. The shape of the premature P wave will look different from that of the sinus P wave on the ECG. The PAC interrupts abruptly. It imposes itself on the normal sinus rhythm (NSR) for one cycle, at which point the SA node resumes control as the dominant pacemaker. PACs are a common phenomenon that do not usually require investigation or treatment.

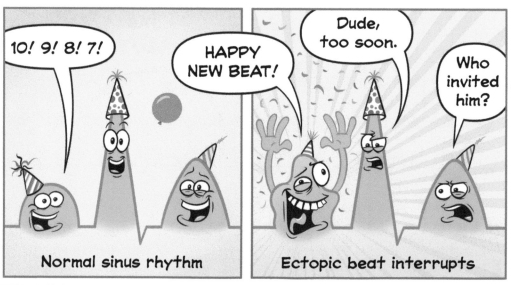

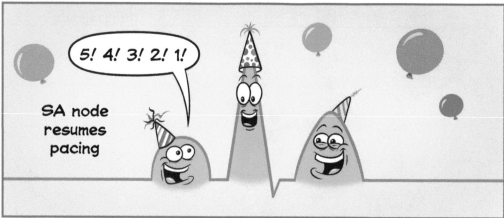

A premature P wave can arrive so early that it becomes superimposed over a wave from the preceding sinus impulse. In this circumstance the premature P wave could be difficult to detect, but careful analysis may reveal a "fusion complex" that is different from all the other waves on the recording. For example, a premature P wave may be embedded on a T wave, making it appear taller than normal.

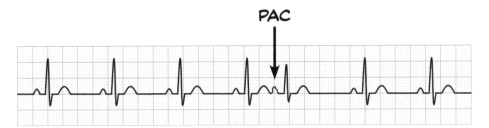

PAC

After an atrial ectopic focus releases an electric impulse, the wave of depolarization also travels in a retrograde fashion to the SA node and "resets" it. The SA node attempts to compensate for the premature beat by creating a pause, but the next cycle with a sinus beat occurs ahead of schedule anyway.

Therefore, the pause is described as being less than compensatory, or more commonly, a *noncompensatory pause*. Each PAC is usually followed by a noncompensatory pause.

QRS is ahead of schedule

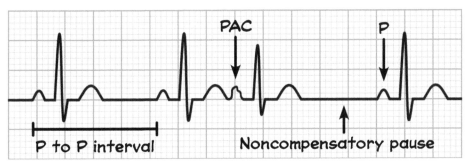

PAC

P

P to P interval

Noncompensatory pause

We can confirm a noncompensatory pause by observing that the P wave following the PAC occurs at less than twice the normal P to P interval. The normal P to P interval can be measured by analyzing the sinus P waves preceding the PAC.

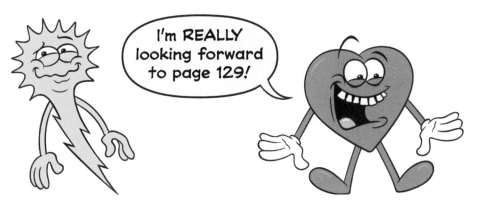

I'm REALLY looking forward to page 129!

If two PACs appear in a row it's called a *couplet*. If three appear in a row, it's called a *triplet*.

A premature atrial complex that arises from a single ectopic focus is classified as a *unifocal* PAC. The PAC looks identical each time it appears.

Premature atrial complexes that arise from two or more ectopic foci are classified as *multifocal* PACs. Each PAC has a different morphology.

Furthermore, PACs often appear in repeating patterns:

- In atrial bigeminy, every other beat is a PAC.
- In atrial trigeminy, every third beat is a PAC.
- In atrial quadrigeminy, every fourth beat is a PAC.

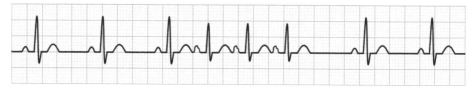

Triplet PACs occur in groups of three

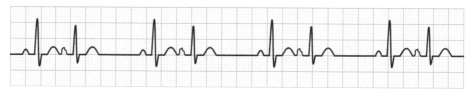

Atrial bigeminy pattern

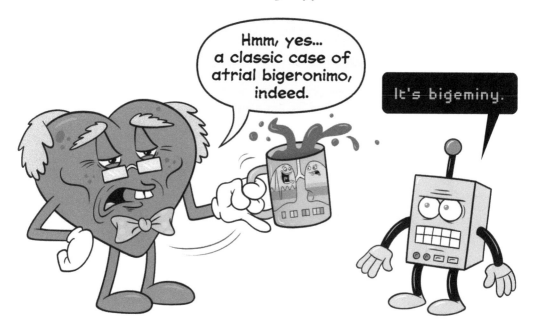

130

Aberrancy occurs when a premature beat causes non-simultaneous depolarization of the ventricles. In this circumstance an ectopic focus fires an impulse when one of the bundle branches is still repolarizing (usually the right bundle branch). One branch is able to receive the impulse from the ectopic focus, but the branch that's repolarizing isn't ready yet because it's still in the refractory period. A delay in conduction occurs, which manifests on the ECG as a widened QRS complex.

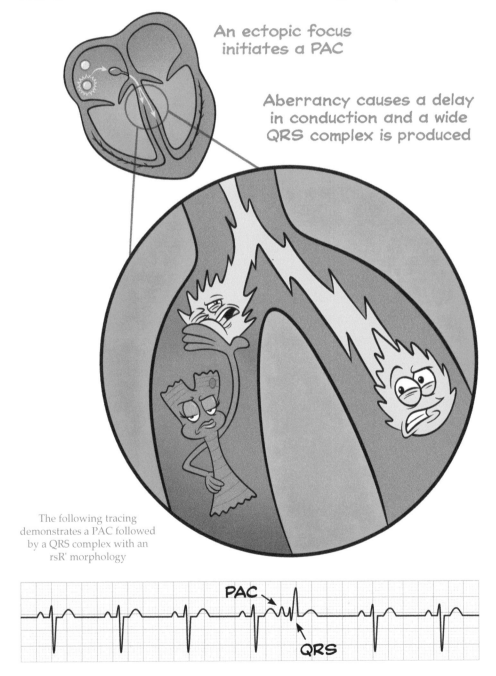

An ectopic focus initiates a PAC

Aberrancy causes a delay in conduction and a wide QRS complex is produced

The following tracing demonstrates a PAC followed by a QRS complex with an rsR' morphology

PAC

QRS

Junctional Premature Beats

Premature beats that arise from an ectopic focus within the AV junction are known as junctional premature beats (JPBs). Like premature atrial complexes, these are common phenomena that are usually of little clinical significance. However, it is possible for PACs or JPBs to provoke other types of arrhythmias.

JPBs are characterized by a premature QRS complex which may be narrow or aberrant. In addition to antegrade conduction, electric impulses firing from the AV junction may also travel backwards to depolarize the atria at any point during ventricular depolarization. This results in upside down waves known as retrograde P waves.

On the ECG, the QRS complex may appear alone as the retrograde P wave is lost in the QRS complex. Alternatively, the retrograde P waves can appear before or after the QRS complex, best seen in leads II, III, and aVF. As with PACs, JPBs can appear as constellations of bigeminy and trigeminy.

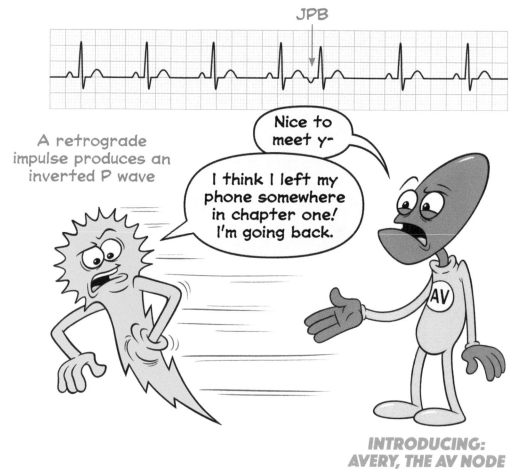

JPB

A retrograde impulse produces an inverted P wave

Nice to meet y-

I think I left my phone somewhere in chapter one! I'm going back.

**INTRODUCING:
AVERY, THE AV NODE**

Paroxysmal Atrial Tachycardia

*Paroxysmal atrial tachycardia (PAT) is usually caused by the sudden activation of an ectopic focus. The underlying mechanism may involve an irritable atrial ectopic focus or a reentry circuit within the atria.

The rate of PAT is 150-250 beats per minute with a regular rhythm. The P waves from PAT have an abnormal appearance because they are generated from outside the SA node. Sometimes the P waves are difficult to detect because they are buried in the preceding T wave.

There is commonly a warm-up phase at the onset of the arrhythmia with gradual shortening of the P to P interval. There may also be a cool-down phase, during which time the rate decelerates with gradual lengthening of the P to P interval. The warm-up and cool-down phases are short, only lasting a few beats.

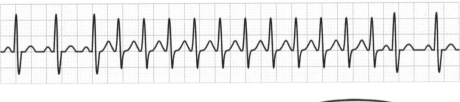

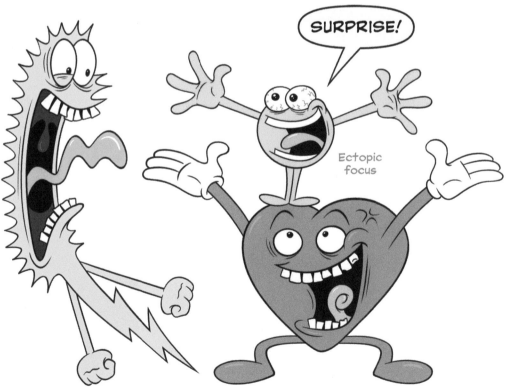

SURPRISE!

Ectopic focus

* Paroxysmal means *sudden*.

Paroxysmal Atrial Tachycardia with Block

PAT with block occurs when an atrial ectopic focus begins pacing rapidly, but the AV node does not transmit its impulses to the ventricles every time. PAT with block is associated with digoxin toxicity. Digoxin may provoke atrial ectopic foci and inhibit the AV node.

The impairment in AV conduction manifests on the ECG as two abnormal P waves for every QRS complex (i.e. a 2:1 ratio of P' waves to QRS complexes). Occasionally the block at the AV node is more severe and a 3:1 ratio is seen.

The atrial rate ranges from 150 to 250 beats per minute. The baseline is isoelectric, and some variation may be seen in the P to P interval. T waves are often indistinguishable from the nonconducted P' waves.

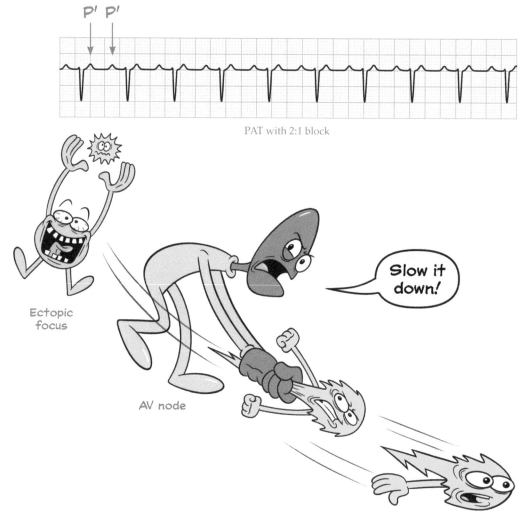

PAT with 2:1 block

Ectopic focus

AV node

Slow it down!

Wandering Atrial Pacemaker

Wandering atrial pacemaker (WAP) is an irregular rhythm produced when pacemaking activity shifts between three or more ectopic foci in the atrial myocardium. The irregular rhythm produces varying cycle lengths with three or more distinct P′ waves.

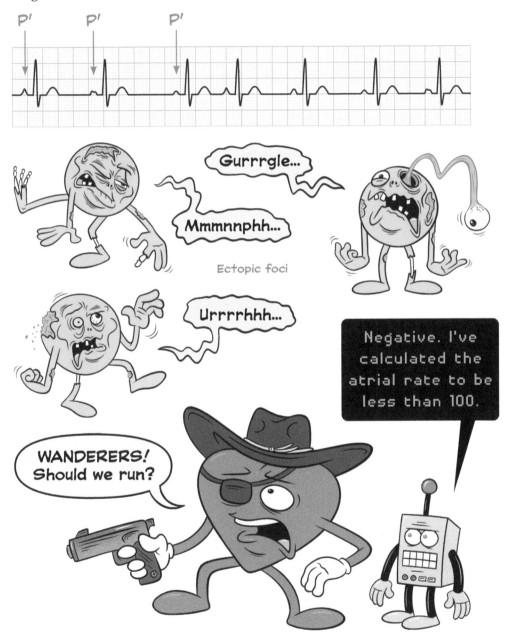

If the rate of WAP accelerates to greater than 100 beats per minute, then the arrhythmia becomes *multifocal atrial tachycardia.*

Multifocal Atrial Tachycardia

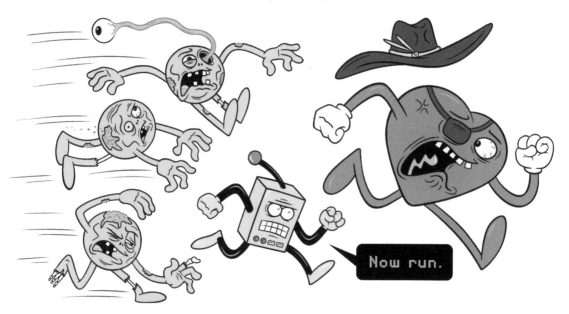

Multifocal atrial tachycardia (MAT) is an irregular rhythm with a rate greater than 100 beats per minute that results from the random firing of three or more ectopic foci. It's like WAP, but faster. Again, P' waves from different sites will demonstrate different morphologies.

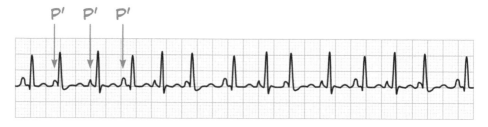

MAT is most commonly seen in patients with chronic obstructive pulmonary disease (COPD). It can also occur with pneumonia, pulmonary embolism, and congestive heart failure.

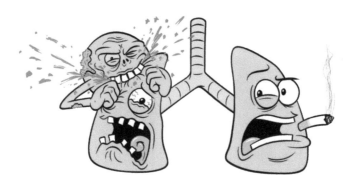

Atrial Flutter

Atrial flutter (AFL) is an extremely rapid rhythm with an atrial rate of 250 to 350 beats per minute. The underlying mechanism of typical atrial flutter is a large reentry circuit usually contained in the right atrium.

On the ECG, atrial flutter produces back-to-back waves known as "flutter" or "F" waves. The rhythm may be regular or irregular. These waves are identical and have a characteristic "sawtooth" appearance. Flutter waves are best seen in leads II, III, and aVF.

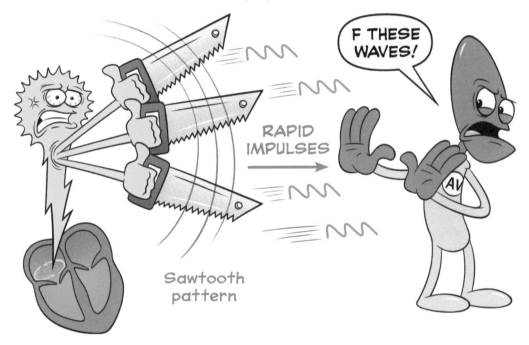

The AV node is bombarded with rapid atrial impulses. Not all impulses are pass through because the AV node needs to repolarize. Electric impulses that reach the AV node during the refractory period are blocked and do not produce a QRS complex. Therefore, the ventricular response rate will vary.

Impulses are most commonly transmitted as a 2:1 AV block, but blocks of 3:1 and 4:1 may also be seen. When in doubt, turning the ECG strip upside down may help identify atrial flutter.

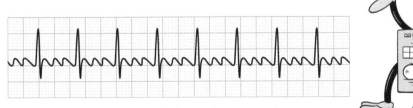

Atrial flutter: rapid atrial rhythm produces sawtooth pattern

Atrial Fibrillation

Atrial fibrillation (AF) is a condition of complete chaos within the atria. The arrhythmia most commonly originates from ectopic foci around the pulmonary vein ostia and may be perpetuated by multiple reentrant circuits throughout the atria. AF is characterized by the absence of P waves on the ECG. Instead, the wild activity from the atria produces a series of irregular oscillations known as fibrillatory waves.

The atria generate between 350 to 600 impulses per minute. The AV node, overwhelmed with the onslaught of atrial impulses, is only able to allow an occasional impulse to pass by. This produces an irregular ventricular rhythm with no set pattern. The absence of any pattern is why atrial fibrillation is often described as being "irregularly irregular."

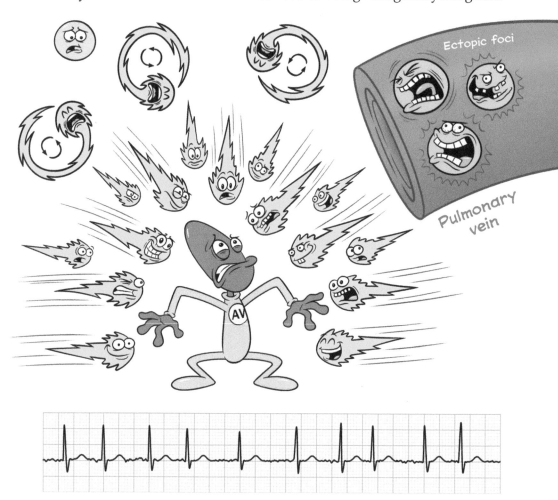

Atrial fibrillation consists of an irregular undulating baseline. The rapid atrial rate produces a variable ventricular response.

AV Nodal Reentry Tachycardia

Atrioventricular nodal reentry tachycardia (AVNRT) is a tachyarrhythmia that develops due to a continuous reentry circuit within the AV node and adjacent atrial myocardium.

The circuit is formed by two pathways that form a loop, namely the slow and fast pathways. The mechanism of the reentry circuit usually involves a premature atrial complex that travels down the slow pathway and then conducts retrograde via the fast pathway, resulting in rapid activation of the ventricles. This is known as "typical" AVNRT.

AVNRT is the most common type of supraventricular tachycardia and typically has a narrow QRS complex. The rate is often between 140 and 280 beats per minute with a regular rhythm. In contrast to paroxysmal atrial tachycardia (PAT), AVNRT does not usually have a warm-up or cool-down period. The rhythm starts and ends abruptly.

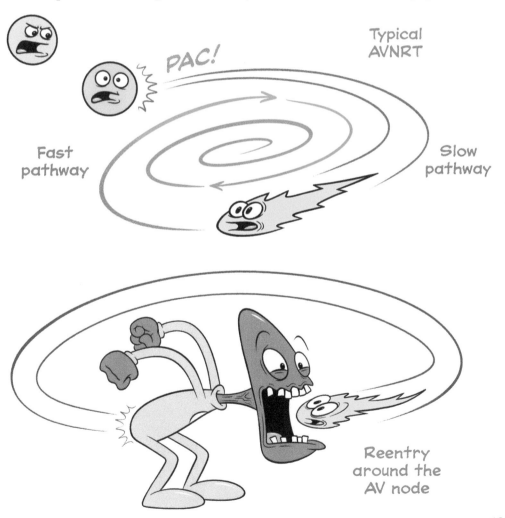

In AVNRT the P′ waves are often embedded within the QRS complexes, which make them difficult to identify.

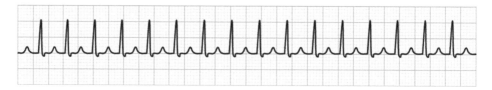

The P′ wave may be superimposed on the end of the QRS complex, producing a *pseudo-R′ wave* in lead V1.

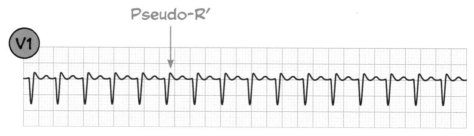

AVNRT: narrow complex tachycardia with regular RR intervals

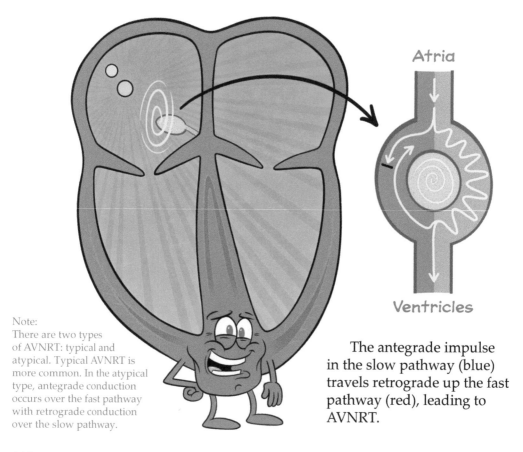

Atria

Ventricles

Note:
There are two types of AVNRT: typical and atypical. Typical AVNRT is more common. In the atypical type, antegrade conduction occurs over the fast pathway with retrograde conduction over the slow pathway.

The antegrade impulse in the slow pathway (blue) travels retrograde up the fast pathway (red), leading to AVNRT.

AV Reciprocating Tachycardia

Atrioventricular reciprocating tachycardia (AVRT), also known as atrioventricular reentrant tachycardia, is a type of SVT that utilizes an accessory bypass tract between the atria and the ventricles to create a continuous circuit with the AV node. It is associated with Wolff-Parkinson-White syndrome. AVRT may be initiated by ectopic beats. The QRS complex can be wide or narrow depending on the direction of electrical conduction. Therefore, there are two main types of AVRT:

- Orthodromic AVRT: antegrade conduction via the AV node with retrograde conduction via the accessory pathway

  - More common form of AVRT

  - Regular, narrow QRS complexes (unless there is a pre-existing bundle branch block or aberrant conduction)

  - Retrograde P' waves may be present

  - May be indistinguishable from AVNRT

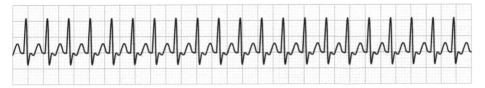

Orthodromic AVRT: narrow complex tachycardia with regular RR intervals

- Antidromic AVRT: antegrade conduction via the accessory pathway with retrograde conduction via the AV node

  - Rare

  - Regular, wide QRS complexes

  - May be difficult to distinguish from ventricular tachycardia

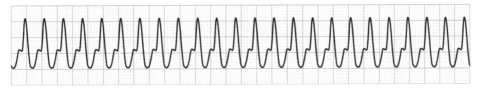

Antidromic AVRT: wide complex tachycardia with regular RR intervals

Narrow Complex Tachycardia

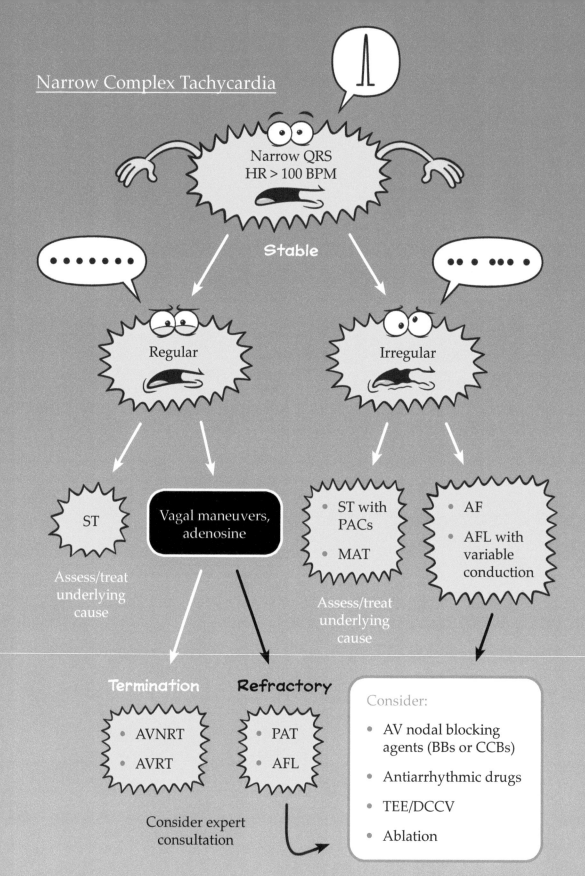

ST: sinus tachycardia, PACs: premature atrial complexes,
MAT: multifocal atrial tachycardia, AF: atrial fibrillation, AFL: atrial flutter,
AVNRT: AV nodal reentry tachycardia, AVRT: AV reciprocating tachycardia

Supraventricular tachycardia

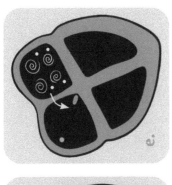
a.

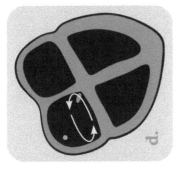
b.

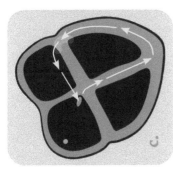
c.

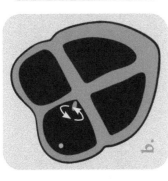
d.

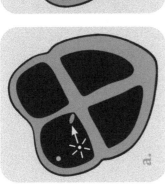
e.

a. Paroxysmal atrial tachycardia (PAT): sudden activation of an ectopic focus with an automatic, triggered, or microreentrant mechanism.

b. AV nodal reentry tachycardia (AVNRT): reentry circuit between the AV node and adjacent atrial myocardium. The circuit involves two pathways: a fast pathway and a slow pathway. Typically, a PAC causes a unidirectional block in the fast pathway. This allows for antegrade conduction down the slow pathway and retrograde conduction up the fast pathway, which activates the reentry circuit.

c. AV reciprocating tachycardia (AVRT): circuit involves the AV node and an accessory bypass tract, most commonly antegrade conduction down the AV node and then retrograde through the accessory bypass tract from the ventricle to the atria.

d. Atrial flutter (AFL): reentry circuit located in the right atrium.

e. Atrial fibrillation (AF): chaotic rhythm with multiple circuits and multiple foci firing at the same time, most commonly originating from the pulmonary vein ostia.

Vagal Maneuvers

Stimulation of the vagus nerve includes techniques such as the Valsalva maneuver and carotid sinus massage. These physical maneuvers activate the parasympathetic nervous system, causing the local release of acetylcholine in the heart.

Vagal maneuvers can help distinguish AVNRT (which is due to a reentry circuit) from other supraventricular arrhythmias such as PAT (which is caused by irritable ectopic foci). For example, carotid sinus massage may terminate AVNRT, but have virtually no effect on PAT.

Therefore, vagal maneuvers can be both diagnostic and therapeutic. Furthermore, vagal maneuvers may be used for an equivocal rhythm. In the case of atrial flutter, initiating a vagal maneuver can increase the AV block to reveal the characteristic flutter waves more clearly.

Carotid sinus massage is often not recommended in the elderly due to the risk of dislodging an atherosclerotic plaque and causing a stroke.

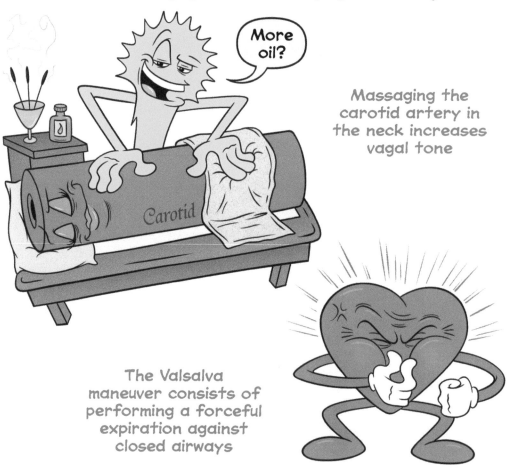

Massaging the carotid artery in the neck increases vagal tone

The Valsalva maneuver consists of performing a forceful expiration against closed airways

Premature Ventricular Complexes

A premature ventricular complex (PVC) is a premature beat produced by an ectopic focus distal to the bifurcation of the bundle of His. PVCs are the most common type of ventricular arrhythmia.

A PVC produces a wide and bizarre QRS complex with a large amplitude. The QRS duration is almost always greater than 0.12 seconds. The T wave is characterized by a deflection in the opposite direction of the major QRS component (e.g. a predominantly positive QRS complex will be followed by an inverted T wave). PVCs aren't usually preceded by P waves, but retrograde depolarization of the atria is possible.

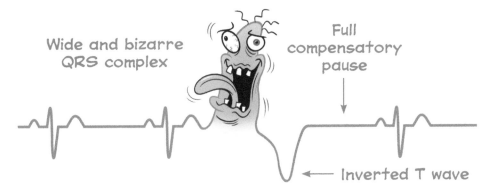

In contrast to PACs, PVCs are usually followed by a **full** compensatory pause in which the timing of the rhythm remains identical before and after the pause. The SA node must remain unaffected by the PVC in order for this to occur (i.e. the SA node is not reset). PVCs can appear randomly or occur in patterns such as bigeminy, trigeminy, and quadrigeminy. They may also appear as couplets or triplets. Most cases of isolated PVCs are a normal phenomenon that rarely require investigation or treatment.

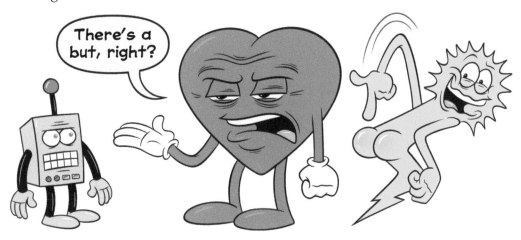

BUT, there are circumstances in which PVCs appear to pose an increased risk for triggering dangerous ventricular arrhythmias. This includes cases of frequent PVCs, a run of three or more consecutive PVCs, PVCs from distinct ectopic foci (so called "multiform" PVCs), and PVCs occurring in the setting of acute myocardial infarction.

Life-threatening ventricular rhythms can also be triggered if a PVC occurs so early that it falls on the T wave of the previous beat. This is known as the *R on T phenomenon*.

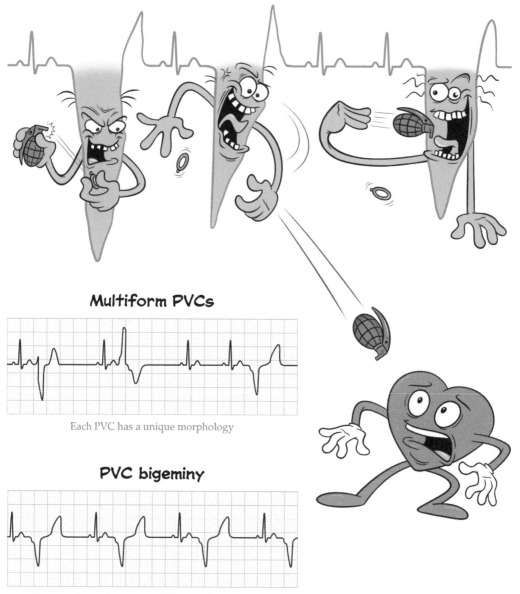

Multiform PVCs

Each PVC has a unique morphology

PVC bigeminy

There is a 1:1 ratio between PVCs and the sinus beats

PVC vs. Ashman Phenomenon

Ashman phenomenon describes a long R to R interval which is immediately followed by a short R to R interval (e.g. that of a premature atrial complex). The supraventricular beat is *aberrantly conducted, producing a wide QRS that resembles a PVC.

The Ashman phenomenon is commonly seen in atrial fibrillation where there are frequent episodes of alternating long and short R to R intervals.

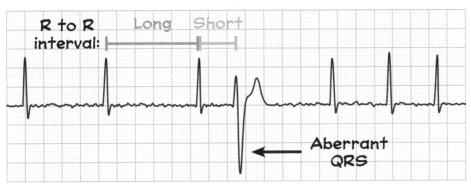

Ashman phenomenon

R to R interval: Long Short

Aberrant QRS

Some tips to distinguish a PVC from Ashman phenomenon:

- The absence of a long and short R to R cycle suggests a PVC.

- A PVC is usually followed by a longer R to R interval due to a full compensatory pause. A heart rate that remains unaltered after the appearance of a wide QRS suggests a PVC.

- Undulation of the baseline due to atrial fibrillation favors an aberrantly conducted supraventricular beat.

- The absence of P waves in a regular rhythm suggests a PVC.

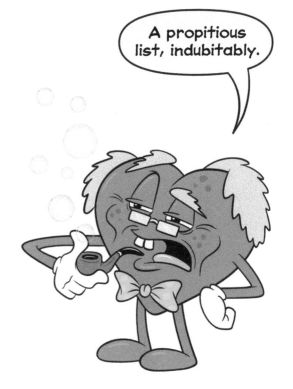

A propitious list, indubitably.

* The concept of aberrancy was introduced on page 131.

Accelerated Idioventricular Rhythm

Accelerated idioventricular rhythm (AIVR) occurs when a ventricular ectopic focus increases its depolarization rate and usurps pacing control from the SA node.

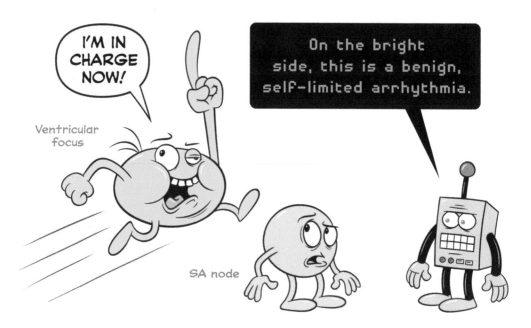

AIVR exists on the ECG when there are three or more consecutive ventricular beats at a regular rhythm at a rate of 50 to 110 beats per minute.

AIVR most commonly occurs in the setting of acute myocardial infarction. It is also a common manifestation of digoxin toxicity. The arrhythmia is considered a benign escape rhythm that can appear when the sinus rate slows and disappear when the sinus rate speeds up. Management of AIVR involves treating the underlying cause.

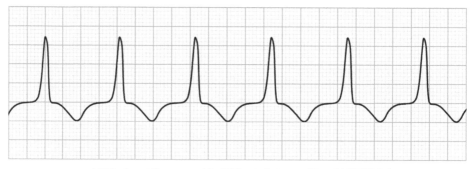

AIVR: absent P waves, wide QRS, rate between 50 and 110 BPM.

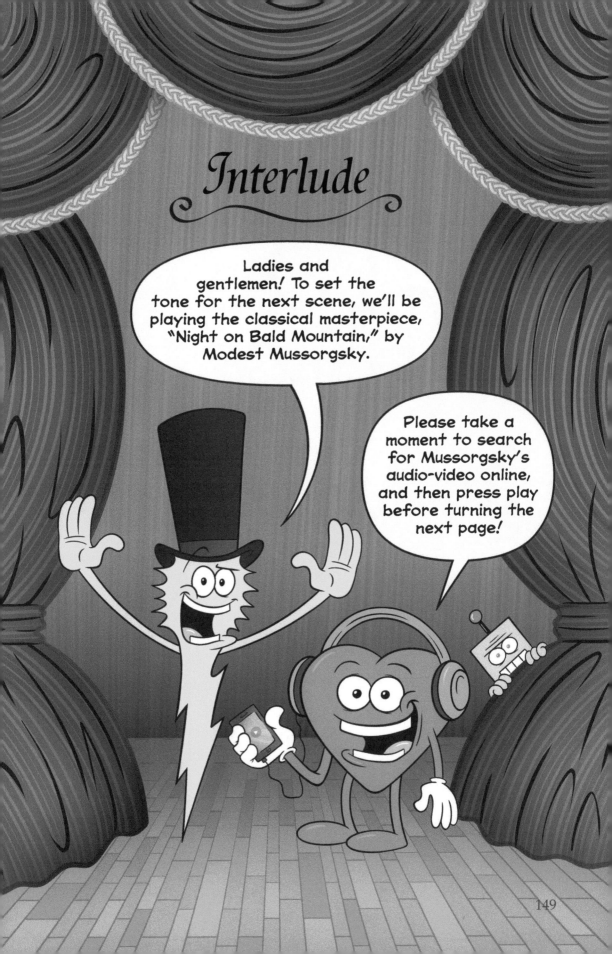

MALIGNANT VENTRICULAR ARRHYTHMIAS

SUSTAINED VENTRICULAR TACHYCARDIA

TORSADES DE POINTES

VENTRICULAR FIBRILLATION

ABNORMAL MYOCARDIAL DEPOLARIZATION

INCREASED RISK OF SUDDEN CARDIAC DEATH

DECREASED CARDIAC OUTPUT

REQUIRE IMMEDIATE MEDICAL ATTENTION

Ventricular Tachycardia

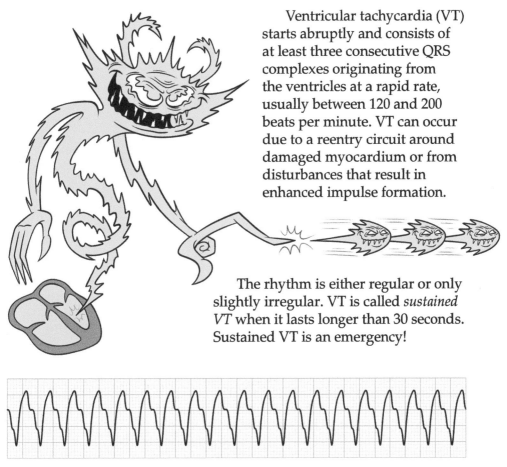

Ventricular tachycardia (VT) starts abruptly and consists of at least three consecutive QRS complexes originating from the ventricles at a rapid rate, usually between 120 and 200 beats per minute. VT can occur due to a reentry circuit around damaged myocardium or from disturbances that result in enhanced impulse formation.

The rhythm is either regular or only slightly irregular. VT is called *sustained VT* when it lasts longer than 30 seconds. Sustained VT is an emergency!

Monomorphic (uniform) VT: each QRS complex is nearly identical

A pacemaker in the atrium usually continues depolarizing independently to the ventricles during VT. These P waves can sometimes be identified as a notch or irregularity on the QRS complexes. *AV dissociation* occurs when the atrial rhythm is independent from the ventricular rhythm. However, the atria can be associated with the ventricles if retrograde depolarization occurs.

The duration of the QRS complex is usually ≥ 0.16 seconds. If the appearance of the QRS complex changes from beat to beat, it is known as *polymorphic VT*.

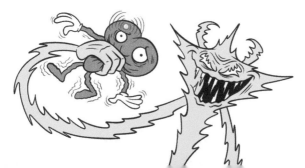

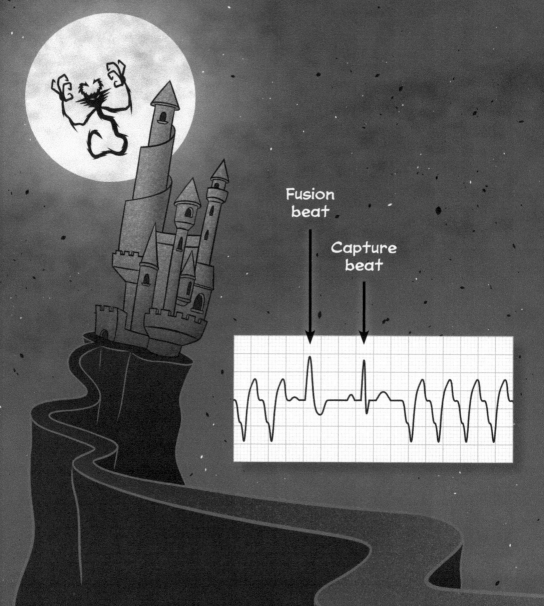

Fusion beat

Capture beat

During VT, a sinus beat will occasionally occur at the same time as a ventricular beat. This produces an intermediate hybrid complex known as a *fusion beat*.

A *capture beat* is another type of beat that can occur in the midst of VT. It describes a sinus beat that occurs at just the right moment to depolarize the ventricles through the cardiac conduction system, resulting in a normal QRS complex.

Two additional features suggestive of VT are Brugada's and Josephson's signs.

Brugada's sign is when the duration from the start of the QRS complex to the bottom of the S wave is > 0.10 seconds.

Josephson's sign represents a small notch near the low point of the S wave.

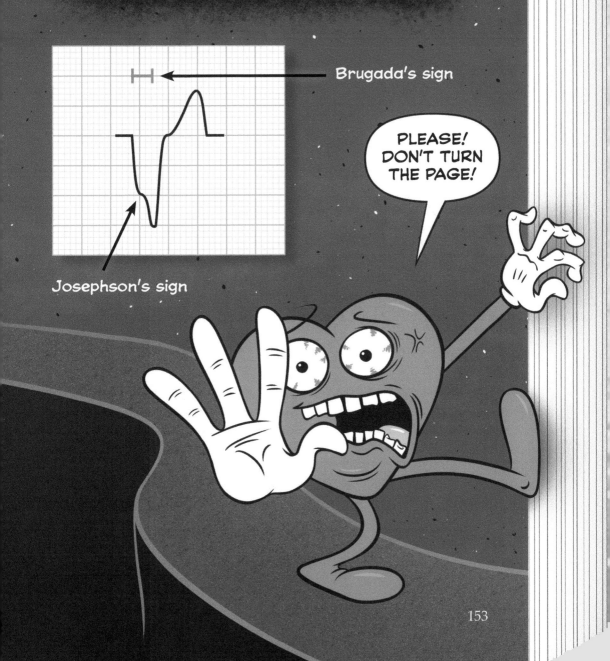

Brugada's sign

Josephson's sign

PLEASE! DON'T TURN THE PAGE!

Torsades De Pointes

Torsades de pointes is a type of polymorphic VT that occurs in the presence of a prolonged QT interval. The name is French for "twisting of the points." It describes the characteristic appearance of the QRS complexes which continuously change shape and amplitude as if twisting around the baseline. The rate generally varies from 200 to 300 beats per minute.

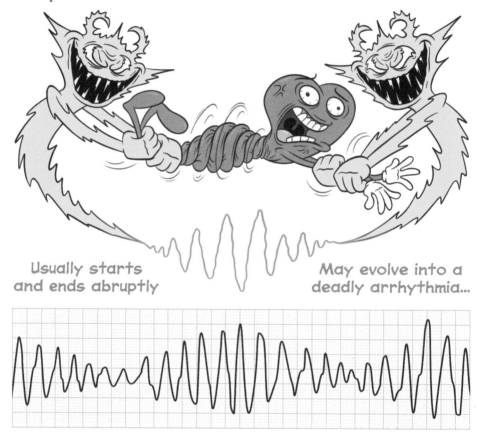

Usually starts and ends abruptly

May evolve into a deadly arrhythmia...

A prolonged QT interval can be caused by antiarrhythmic drugs (e.g. quinidine, procainamide, sotalol, disopyramide), macrolide antibiotics, some antifungals, and tricyclic antidepressants, among many other agents. It is also caused by electrolyte disturbances (e.g. hypokalemia, hypomagnesemia, hypocalcemia), or occur in the setting of acute myocardial infarction or stroke. QT prolongation may also be congenital in origin as seen in *long QT syndrome (LQTS)*.

QT prolongation represents an increase in the time it takes for the ventricles to repolarize. This means that the T wave is also lengthened, making it more likely that a PVC could fall on the elongated T wave and set off torsades de pointes (R on T phenomenon).

Ventricular Fibrillation

The most dangerous ventricular arrhythmia is ventricular fibrillation (VF), which can cause death within minutes. In VF the ventricles attempt to contract at a rate of up to 500 times per minute. This causes the heart to quiver chaotically and lose its function as an effective pump (i.e. there is a complete loss of cardiac output).

During VF the ECG will show erratic deflections of varying shape and amplitude. When the fibrillatory waves are large the ECG tracing is described as "coarse" ventricular fibrillation. Small fibrillatory waves characterize "fine" ventricular fibrillation, which can degenerate to asystole.

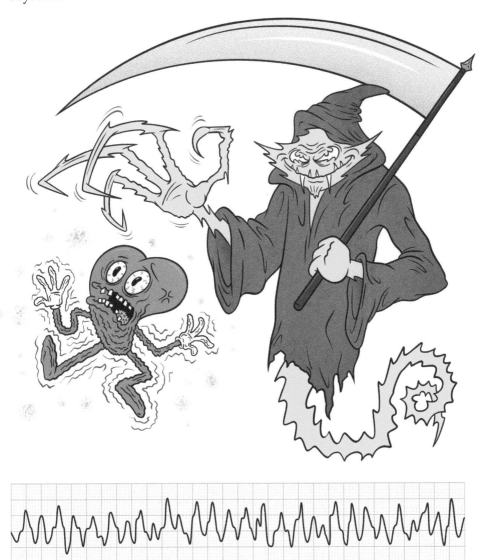

Defibrillation

Ventricular fibrillation and pulseless ventricular tachycardia are non-perfusing rhythms. The single most important treatment modality for these arrhythmias is defibrillation, which involves the delivery of an electric shock across the heart in an attempt to convert the arrhythmia to normal sinus rhythm.

A convenient way to perform defibrillation is with the use of an automated external defibrillator (AED). This portable electronic device is widely available in many public venues. It comes equipped with electrode pads that attach to the external chest wall. The AED is able to automatically analyze the heart's rhythm and deliver life-saving shocks if necessary.

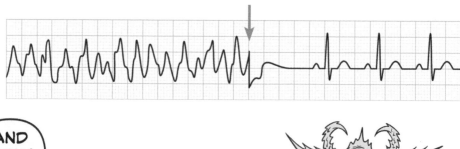

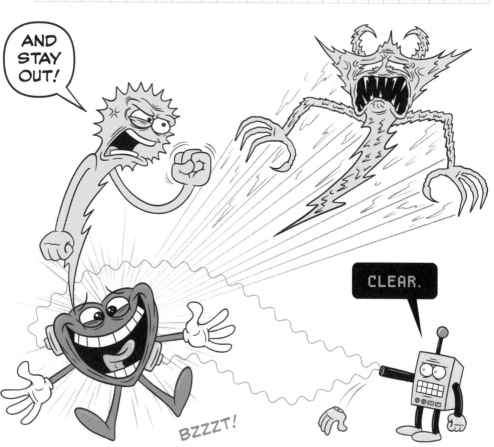

Electrophysiology Studies

Electrophysiology studies (EPS) are minimally invasive tests performed in an electrophysiology laboratory to assess the function of the heart's electrical conduction system.

The studies are performed by introducing catheters that contain electrodes through the peripheral veins or arteries, and into various locations within the heart.

In general, EPS are most often recommended for patients with recurrent episodes of documented or highly suspected symptomatic arrhythmias (e.g. symptomatic sustained VT, Stokes-Adams syndrome).

During an EP study, the efficacy of antiarrhythmic drugs may be tested on the heart. In addition, arrhythmias are provoked in order to assess the flow of electricity during actual events. The data from the study can then be analyzed to potentially reveal the origin of an arrhythmia within the heart.

EPS help guide the treatment for an underlying arrhythmia, including options such as antiarrhythmic medications, pacemaker or implantable cardioverter defibrillator (ICD) implantation, cardiac ablation, or surgery.

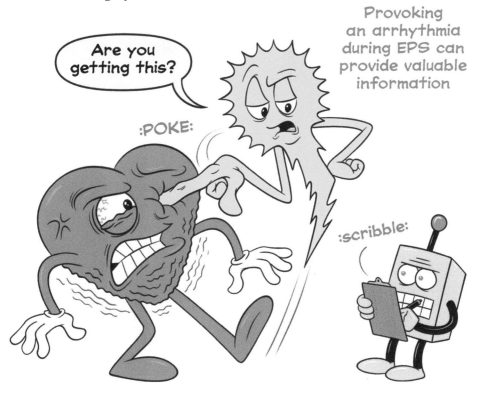

Implantable Cardioverter Defibrillator

The implantable cardioverter defibrillator (ICD) is a small electronic device that provides continuous monitoring of the heart for life-threatening arrhythmias.

ICD placement is typically indicated for patients with a prior episode of ventricular fibrillation or ventricular tachycardia, as well as primary prevention in patients considered to be at high risk for developing malignant ventricular arrhythmias.

The ICD is usually implanted subcutaneously on the chest, with wire leads that are threaded transvenously into the right side of the heart.

The ICD is programmed to distinguish between arrhythmias that require intervention and provide the appropriate treatment. For example, it can institute a shock during ventricular tachycardia to bring the heart back to normal sinus rhythm, initiate overdrive suppression to treat tachyarrhythmias, or provide pacing beats if the heart suddenly becomes bradycardic.

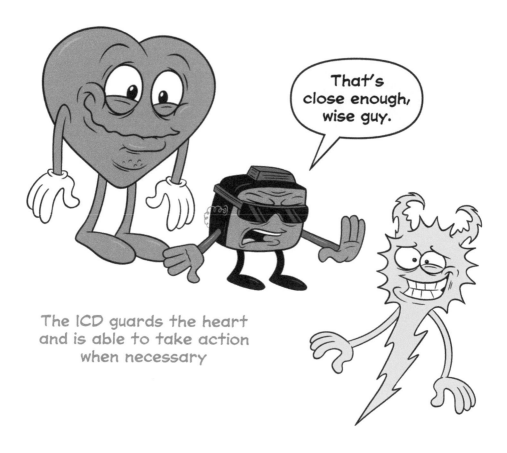

The ICD guards the heart and is able to take action when necessary

Sparkson's Summary: Chapter 7

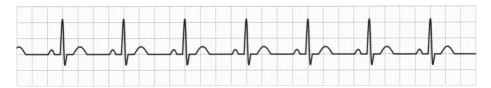

Normal sinus rhythm: sinus rhythm between 60 and 100 beats per minute

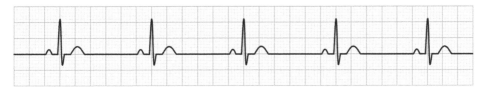

Sinus bradycardia: sinus rhythm less than 60 beats per minute

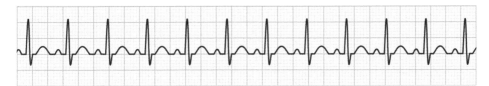

Sinus tachycardia: sinus rhythm greater than 100 beats per minute

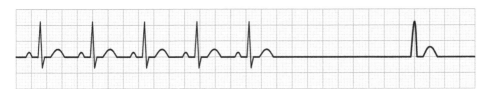

Sinus arrest: SA node fails to depolarize, resulting in prolonged absence of a P wave

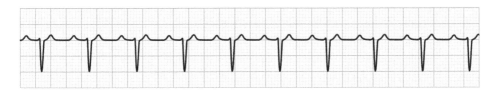

PAT with block: rapid ectopic atrial rhythm with variable conduction to ventricles

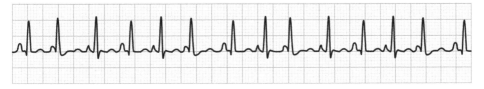

MAT: irregular tachyarrhythmia produced by three or more atrial ectopic foci

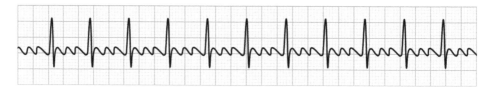

Atrial flutter: rapid atrial rhythm produces sawtooth pattern with variable ventricular response

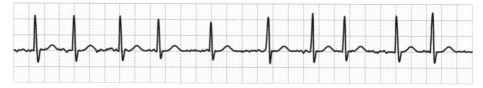

Atrial fibrillation: irregularly irregular rhythm with undulating baseline and absent P waves

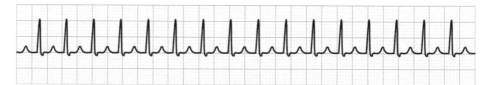

AVNRT: narrow complex tachycardia with regular RR intervals (AVRT may be indistinguishable)

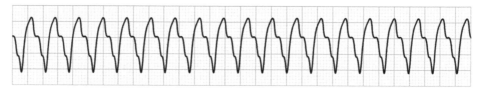

Ventricular tachycardia: wide complex tachycardia originating from the ventricles

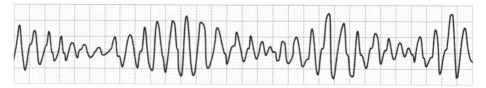

Torsades de pointes: polymorphic VT which may occur in the setting of QT prolongation

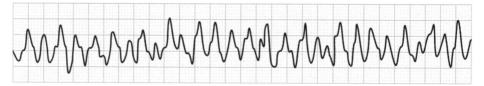

Ventricular fibrillation: erratic ventricular rhythm of varying shape and amplitude

CHAPTER 8

PREEXCITATION AND BLOCKS

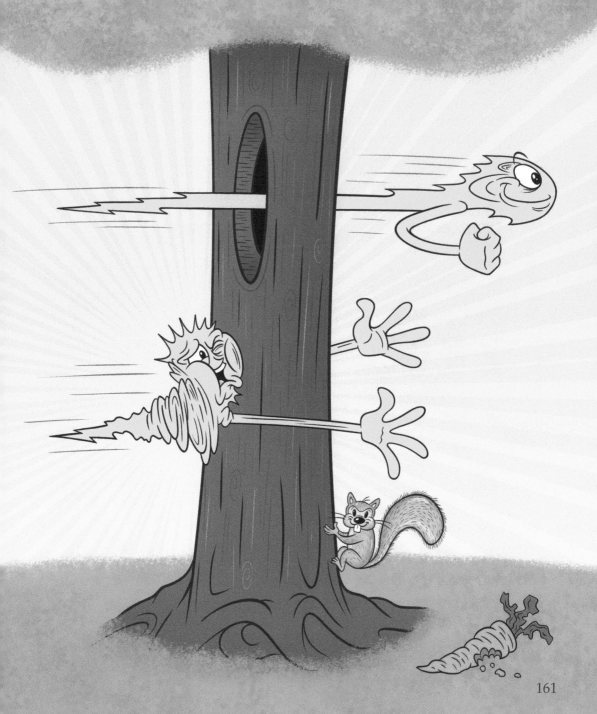

Preexcitation Syndromes

In the preexcitation syndromes, electric impulses bypass a part of the normal cardiac conduction system through an alternative congenital pathway called an "accessory" pathway. The two major preexcitation syndromes are Wolff-Parkinson-White (WPW) syndrome and Lown-Ganong-Levine (LGL) syndrome.

The accessory pathway conducts impulses to the ventricles faster than normal, which shortens the PR interval to less than 0.12 seconds. Furthermore, the accessory pathway can also function as an anatomic reentry circuit, predisposing the heart to tachyarrhythmias.

The most common tachyarrhythmias associated with the preexcitation syndromes are *atrioventricular reentry tachycardia (AVRT) and atrial fibrillation.

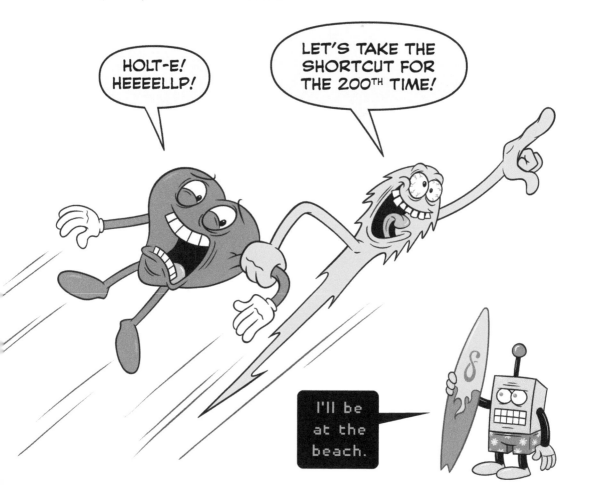

* Not to be confused with AVNRT, found on page 139. The reentry circuit in AVNRT involves the AV node and a small area of the adjacent atrial myocardium. In contrast, AVRT utilizes the AV node-His-Purkinje system along with an accessory pathway to engage in a reentry circuit.

Wolff-Parkinson-White Syndrome

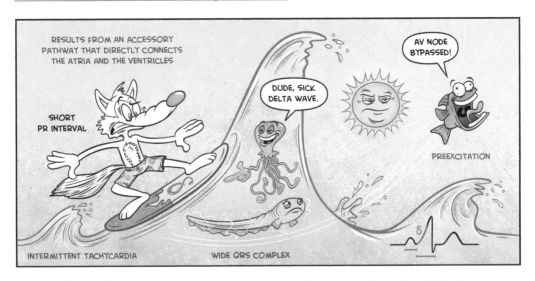

In WPW, the accessory pathway is referred to as the bundle of Kent, which directly connects the atria to the ventricles. The accessory pathway can be found on the left or right side of the heart. Depolarization through the bundle of Kent prematurely "excites" the ventricles, which produces a slurred upstroke on the QRS complex called a *delta wave*.

The PR interval, which represents the time from the start of atrial depolarization to the start of ventricular depolarization, is shortened to less than 0.12 seconds. In addition, the QRS complex is widened to greater than 0.11 seconds. To summarize, the characteristic features of WPW on the ECG include a short PR interval, wide QRS complex, and the presence of a delta wave.

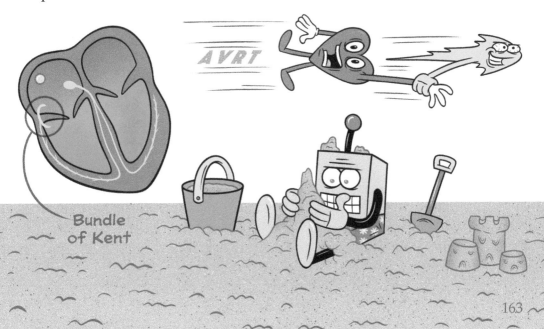

Lown-Ganong-Levine Syndrome

Lown-Ganong-Levine (LGL) syndrome consists of a short PR interval, normal QRS duration, and episodes of tachycardia. In LGL syndrome, the accessory pathway is referred to as the James bundle (or James fibers).

The underlying cause for the short PR interval is unclear, but the most likely explanation is the existence of an intranodal bypass tract. This theory describes a fast pathway directly through the AV node which skips the delay that the electric impulse normally encounters.

Another mechanism for LGL syndrome has been described which postulates the existence of a tract that connects the atrial myocardium directly to the bundle of His. This accessory pathway bypasses the AV node, thus reducing the PR interval to less than 0.12 seconds.

From the bundle of His, the electric impulse can complete the usual cardiac conduction route to depolarize the ventricles normally. Therefore, there is no delta wave and the QRS complex is not widened as in WPW.

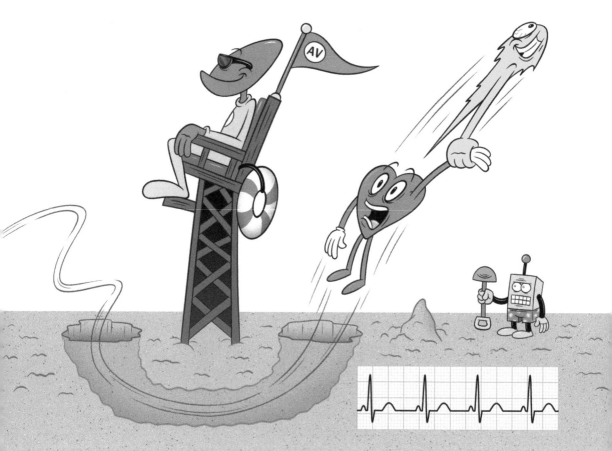

Let's review the path of normal cardiac conduction before continuing on our journey.

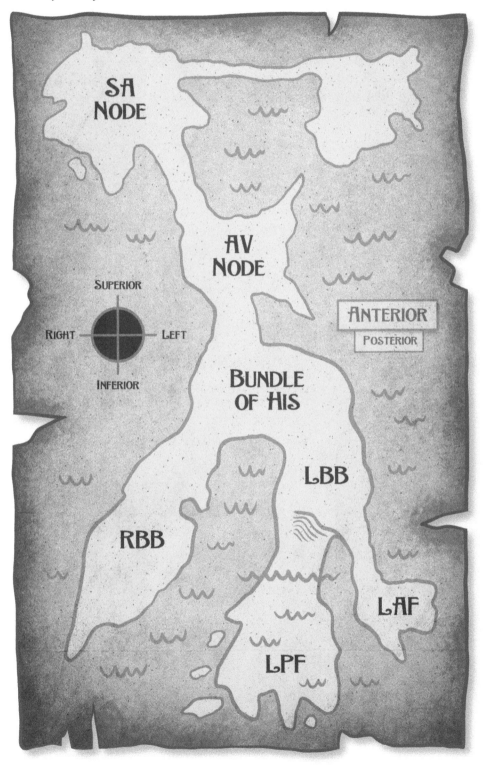

Blocks

A block is any obstruction or delay in the normal cardiac conduction system. Blocks can occur along any electrical pathway in the heart. We already discussed one type of block on page 126 called sinoatrial exit block. In this chapter we'll take a look at blocks that affect the distal conduction system such as atrioventricular (AV) blocks, bundle branch blocks, and fascicular blocks (previously known as hemiblocks).

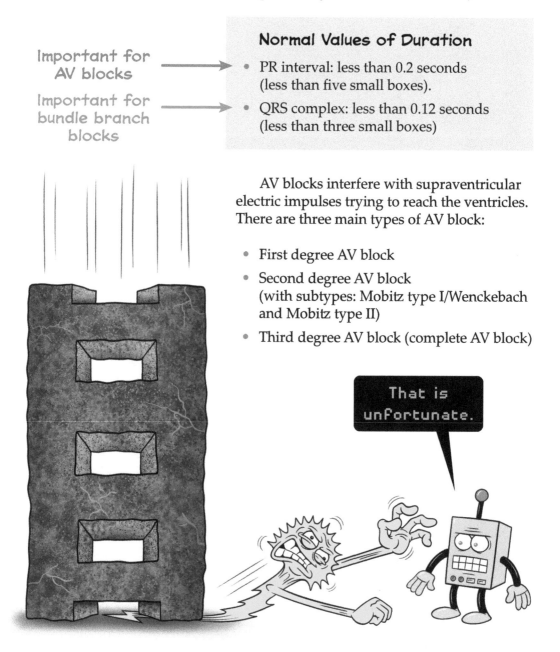

Important for AV blocks

Important for bundle branch blocks

Normal Values of Duration

- PR interval: less than 0.2 seconds (less than five small boxes).

- QRS complex: less than 0.12 seconds (less than three small boxes)

AV blocks interfere with supraventricular electric impulses trying to reach the ventricles. There are three main types of AV block:

- First degree AV block
- Second degree AV block (with subtypes: Mobitz type I/Wenckebach and Mobitz type II)
- Third degree AV block (complete AV block)

First-degree AV Block

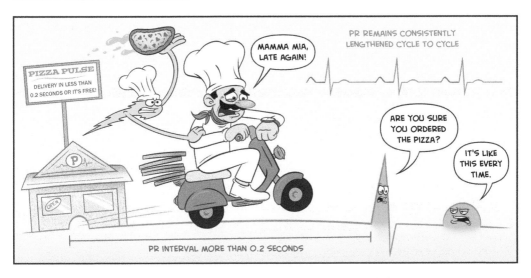

First-degree AV block is characterized by a PR interval that remains consistently lengthened from cycle to cycle. The PR interval represents the time from the start of atrial depolarization to the start of ventricular depolarization.

Each electric impulse from the atria experiences a prolonged delay at the AV node or bundle of His as it makes its way to the ventricles. Despite the delay, each electric impulse does manage to eventually reach the ventricles with a regular rate and rhythm.

The delay in first-degree AV block is defined as a PR interval longer than 0.2 seconds, or five small boxes.

First-degree AV block may occur in healthy individuals as a normal variant. It may also be associated with certain drugs (e.g. digoxin, beta blockers, calcium channel blockers, amiodarone), myocardial infarction, or other disease processes.

No treatment is generally needed for first-degree AV block.

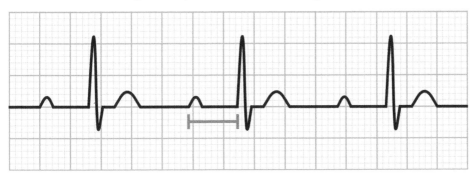

Second-degree AV Blocks

In a second-degree AV block some atrial impulses are conducted, but others are not. Unlike first-degree AV block, not every impulse is able to pass the AV node to reach the ventricles. There are two types of second-degree AV block, termed Mobitz type I (also known as Wenckebach) and Mobitz type II.

Mobitz Type I Second-degree AV Block (Wenckebach)

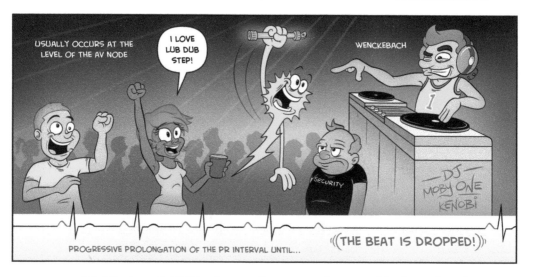

Mobitz type I AV block usually occurs due to a block within the AV node. It is characterized by progressive prolongation of the PR interval until an atrial impulse is completely blocked (the beat is dropped).

The last P wave in the series will appear without the company of a QRS complex because the atrial impulse failed to reach the ventricles.

The sequence repeats itself over and over, with the QRS complex usually dropping every third or fourth beat. Therefore, the series has a consistent P to QRS ratio such as 3:2 or 4:3 (one less QRS complex than the number of P waves in a sequence).

The risk of progression to a more dangerous arrhythmia is generally low and pacemaker insertion is not usually required.

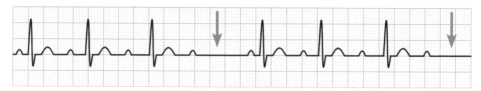

Mobitz type I AV block: progressive prolongation of the PR interval until a QRS complex is dropped

Mobitz Type II Second-degree AV Block

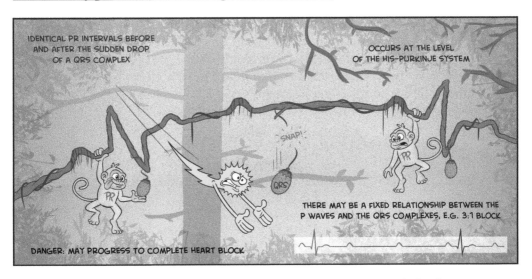

Mobitz type II AV block, which is less common than Wenckebach, usually occurs from a block below the AV node at the level of the His-Purkinje system.

It differs from Wenckebach in that there is no progressive lengthening of the PR interval. Instead, Mobitz type II is characterized by identical PR intervals before and after non-conducted atrial beats.

Therefore, Mobitz type II is referred to as an "all or nothing" phenomenon, in which the His-Purkinje cells suddenly fail to conduct an atrial impulse. The series then repeats.

The block may demonstrate a fixed relationship between the P waves and QRS complexes such as 2:1 (two P waves for every one QRS) or 3:1 (three P waves for every one QRS). Alternatively, the block may not consist of any identifiable pattern.

Mobitz type II AV block is a serious problem with the potential to progress to the extremely dangerous third degree AV block. Thus, treatment for Mobitz type II often requires permanent artificial pacemaker insertion.

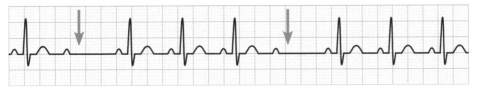

Mobitz type II AV block: the PR interval does not lengthen before or after the dropped QRS complex

Distinguishing 2:1 Wenckebach from 2:1 Mobitz Type II

When the AV conduction ratio is 2:1 (i.e. two P waves for every one QRS complex), it may be impossible to determine whether the pattern is due to a Wenckebach block or due to a Mobitz type II block. Wenckebach block involves progressive lengthening of the PR interval, but with the QRS complex dropping so frequently we do not get enough PR intervals in one sequence to make that determination.

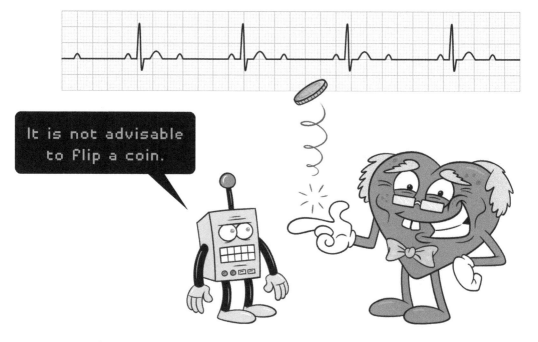

It is not advisable to flip a coin.

Why is it important to make the distinction? While the Wenckebach block represents a relatively benign process, Mobitz type II is a dangerous and potentially life-threatening arrhythmia.

An extended period of observation can help in the diagnosis. This includes techniques such as obtaining a long rhythm strip, watching a cardiac monitor, or obtaining serial ECGs. The goal with these approaches is to record a change in the conduction ratio which would reveal the behavior of the PR interval.

Another option is to employ bedside vagal maneuvers. Wenckebach block occurs within the AV node, which is richly supplied with parasympathetic fibers. Therefore, vagal maneuvers could increase the Wenckebach ratio and make the rhythm easier to analyze.

In contrast, a Mobitz type II AV block occurs below the AV node. In this case vagal maneuvers would either have no effect on the block or may eliminate the block and produce 1:1 AV conduction.

Third-degree AV Block

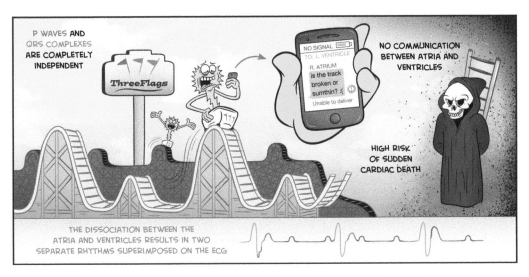

THE DISSOCIATION BETWEEN THE ATRIA AND VENTRICLES RESULTS IN TWO SEPARATE RHYTHMS SUPERIMPOSED ON THE ECG

In third-degree AV block, also known as complete heart block, none of the atrial impulses are able to reach the ventricles. The risk of sudden cardiac death is high as the ventricles are no longer able to rely on the atria to initiate ventricular depolarization.

In order for the heart to maintain a perfusing rhythm, an ectopic focus below the level of the block escapes and assumes pacing responsibility at its inherent rate. This is called the *idioventricular escape rhythm*.

Third-degree AV block always produces AV dissociation, which results in two separate rhythms superimposed on the ECG tracing. The atria usually continue to contract at a regular rate, producing P waves completely independent to the slower QRS complex rate.

Complete heart block can cause Stokes-Adams syndrome or sudden cardiac death and the condition almost always requires the insertion of a permanent artificial pacemaker.

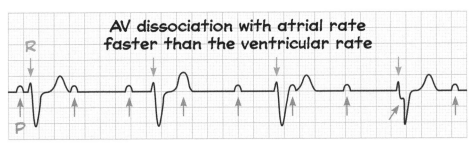

Third-degree AV block: P waves march along at their own rate, wide QRS complexes suggest a ventricular origin

Third-degree AV block can occur at the level of the AV node or lower. If it occurs at the level of the AV node, the condition is typically less severe because a junctional ectopic focus is able to escape and pace the heart at its inherent rate of 40 to 60 beats per minute (BPM). This activity produces a narrow QRS complex due to its location above the ventricles.

If third-degree AV block occurs at a lower level (e.g. in the ventricles), it is likely to produce a wide QRS complex with a very slow escape rate. This type of third-degree AV block is extremely dangerous.

Causes of third-degree AV block include myocardial infarction, AV-nodal blocking medications (calcium channel blockers, beta blockers, digoxin), Lyme disease, and idiopathic degeneration of the conduction system.

Third-degree AV block with a ventricular focus

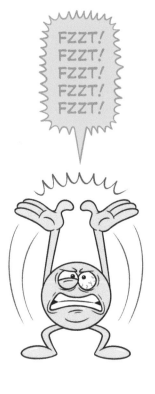

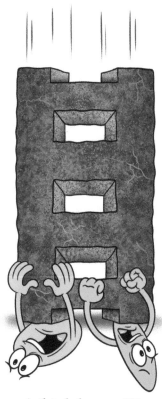

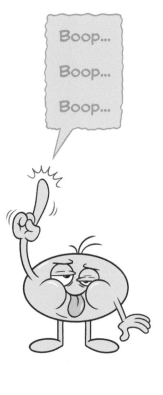

Depolarizations from the SA node continue, but none are able to reach the ventricles

A third-degree AV block below the level of the AV node inhibits pacing activity from atrial or junctional ectopic foci

A ventricular focus assumes responsibility and provides a rescue rhythm at its inherent rate (20 to 40 BPM)

Bundle Branch Blocks

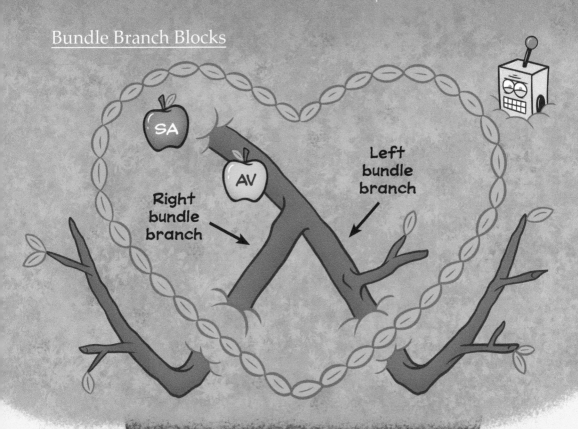

A bundle branch block is a conduction block in the right or left bundle branch. It causes a significant delay in conduction to the affected ventricle. Thus, a bundle branch block does not necessarily imply complete transmission failure.

The QRS complex, which represents ventricular depolarization, is widened on the ECG because the bundle branch block causes the process of depolarization to take longer than usual.

A normal QRS complex is less than 0.12 seconds in duration.

A bundle branch block is diagnosed by analyzing the duration and morphology of the QRS complex, best seen in the precordial leads. A bundle branch block can also cause repolarization abnormalities such as ST segment depression and T wave inversion.

Right Bundle Branch Block

A right bundle branch block (RBBB) results in delayed conduction through the right bundle branch, but conduction through the left bundle branch remains unaffected. The delay causes the QRS complex to widen to a duration greater than 0.12 seconds.

When a RBBB is present depolarization of the right ventricle occurs slightly later than depolarization of the left ventricle. The asynchronous depolarization of the ventricles produces a characteristic change in the shape of the QRS complex, best seen in leads V1 and V2. These leads record electrical activity over the right ventricle.

We might expect the ventricles to produce separate QRS complexes if they are not depolarizing at the same time. This is technically the case, but the complexes appear superimposed over one another, creating a wide QRS fusion complex that has *two* R waves (two peaks). This is sometimes referred to as the "rabbit ear" or "M" pattern on the ECG.

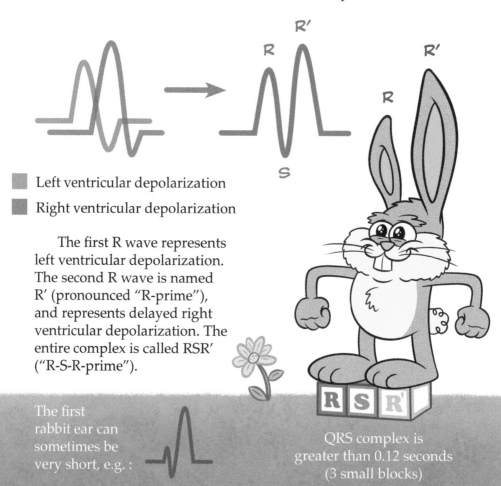

Left ventricular depolarization

Right ventricular depolarization

The first R wave represents left ventricular depolarization. The second R wave is named R' (pronounced "R-prime"), and represents delayed right ventricular depolarization. The entire complex is called RSR' ("R-S-R-prime").

The first rabbit ear can sometimes be very short, e.g. :

QRS complex is greater than 0.12 seconds (3 small blocks)

Delayed activation of the right ventricle may produce downsloping ST segments and T wave inversions in the right precordial leads.

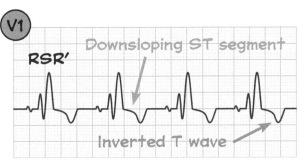

V1

RSR′

Downsloping ST segment

Inverted T wave

Right bundle branch block will also produce wide, slurred S waves in the lateral leads (I, aVL, V5, V6).

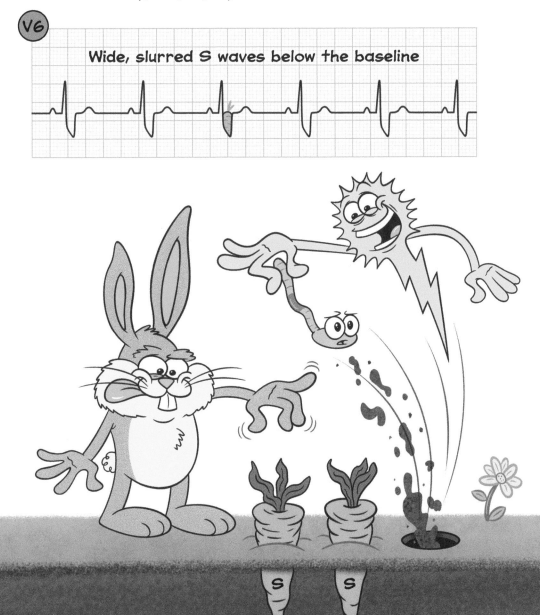

V6

Wide, slurred S waves below the baseline

Left Bundle Branch Block

In left bundle branch block (LBBB) conduction through the left bundle branch is delayed. The right ventricle is activated before the left ventricle and the QRS complex widens beyond 0.12 seconds in duration (3 small boxes). The appearance of the QRS complex is also affected, with the characteristic shape of the QRS complex consisting of a broad, notched top or slurred R wave. In addition, the ST segments and T waves deflect in the direction opposite to the major deflection of the QRS complex.

The changes in morphology of the QRS complex are best seen in leads which record electrical activity over the left ventricle (I, aVL, V5, and V6). Reciprocal changes are seen in leads over the right side of the heart (V1, V2, and V3), consisting of broad, deep S waves. The overall direction of depolarization in LBBB is from right to left, which variably results in left axis deviation.

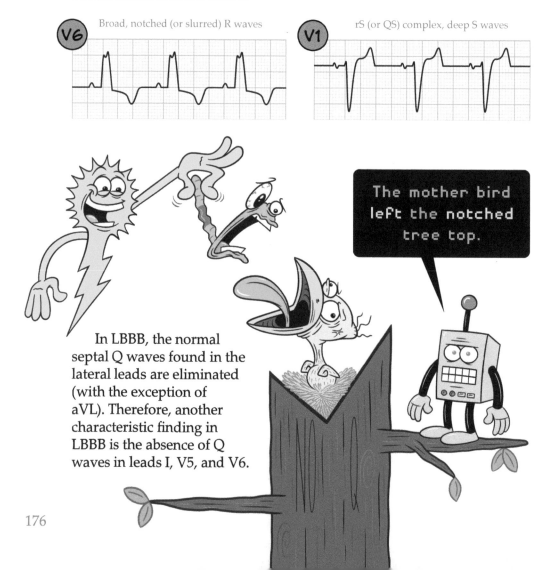

In LBBB, the normal septal Q waves found in the lateral leads are eliminated (with the exception of aVL). Therefore, another characteristic finding in LBBB is the absence of Q waves in leads I, V5, and V6.

Incomplete Bundle Branch Block

An incomplete bundle branch block refers to a conduction abnormality which results in a right or left bundle branch block pattern, but without significant widening of the QRS complex. For example, the rabbit ears of RBBB may be seen in lead V1, but with a QRS duration between 0.10 to 0.12 seconds. The etiologies of incomplete bundle branch blocks are generally the same as those of other bundle branch blocks, but possibly with less clinical significance.

Causes of Bundle Branch Block and NICD

Bundle branch blocks can be idiopathic or associated with a wide variety of disorders. RBBB is fairly common in apparently normal hearts, but can also be caused by myocardial ischemia, infarction, or inflammation. RBBB is also associated with cor pulmonale and pulmonary embolism.

LBBB is associated with underlying heart disease more often than RBBB. It may indicate the presence of ischemic heart disease, progressive degeneration of the cardiac conduction system, hyperkalemia, or digoxin toxicity, among others.

Another type of block, termed a *non-specific intraventricular conduction delay* (NICD), is said to occur when the QRS duration is prolonged to greater than 0.12 seconds, but the criteria for RBBB or LBBB are not met. NICD is a non-specific marker of cardiac pathology.

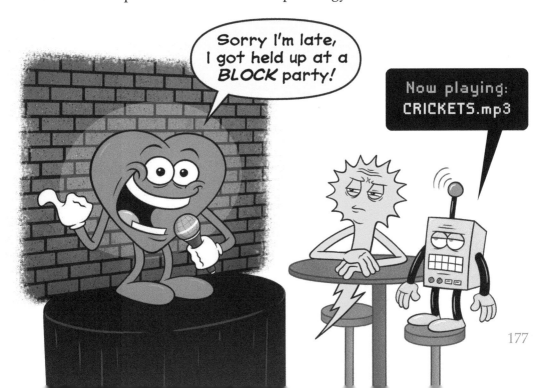

Transient Bundle Branch Block

Transient (intermittent) bundle branch block may have several mechanisms. One such mechanism is a phase 3 block, in which conduction down a bundle branch is blocked because the cells have not had enough time to repolarize. The electric impulse arrives at the bundle branch during the relative refractory period, resulting in a delay. Remember page 6?

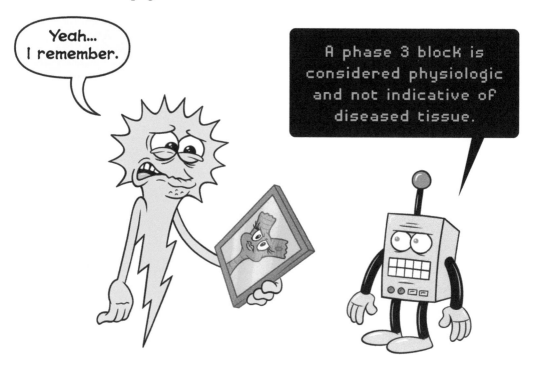

Transient bundle branch block can also occur as an acceleration-dependent block. The bundle branch block only appears if the heart rate increases and reaches a certain threshold. The rate at which the bundle branch block reveals itself is called the *critical rate*. This finding is a manifestation of a diseased His-Purkinje system.

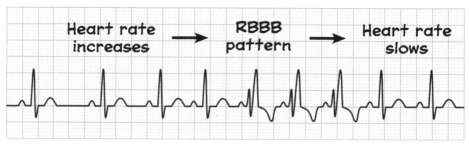

Acceleration-dependent block: RBBB pattern appears when the heart rate accelerates to the critical rate. The block resolves when the heart rate slows below the critical rate

Idiopathic Bundle Branch Block

Idiopathic bundle branch block is characterized by two overlapping syndromes known as *Lenegre's disease* and *Lev's disease*. The names are sometimes used interchangeably or in conjunction (e.g. Lev-Lenegre).

Lenegre's disease mainly refers to a sclerodegenerative disease of the conduction system that tends to affect younger patients. It may be hereditary and carries a risk of progression to complete heart block.

Lev's disease traditionally refers to fibrosis and calcification of the cardiac skeleton in older patients. It usually affects the mitral and aortic annuli, which are the ring-shaped structures that support the valvular leaflets. Conduction blocks can develop when the disease spreads into the cardiac conduction system.

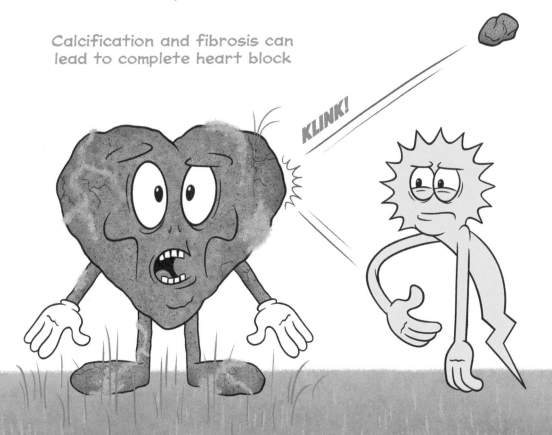

Calcification and fibrosis can lead to complete heart block

KLINK!

Fascicular Blocks

The left bundle branch divides into two major fascicles. These are known as the left anterior fascicle (LAF) and the left posterior fascicle (LPF). A fascicular block is a conduction block along one of these fascicles. I've taken the artistic liberty of illustrating the LAF in a superior position and the LPF in an inferior position to help us visualize the flow of electricity through the fascicles. However, keep in mind that the heart is three dimensional structure with a complex array of Purkinje fibers and the following diagrams represent theoretical simplifications.

As a side note, the left bundle branch also gives way to a third fascicle which supplies the interventricular septum called the septal fascicle, but it is not relevant in our discussion of fascicular blocks. The right bundle branch doesn't have any established subdivisions.

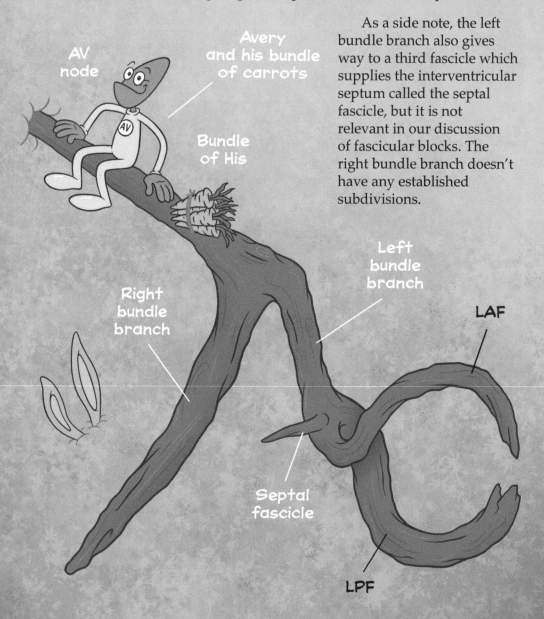

When we learned about right and left bundle branch blocks, focus was placed on the precordial leads to make the diagnosis. However, with fascicular blocks our attention should be drawn to the limb leads. This is important because the diagnosis of a fascicular block completely depends on a change in the ECG's axis. The schematic used to measure axis deviation, the hexaxial reference system, only utilizes limb leads.

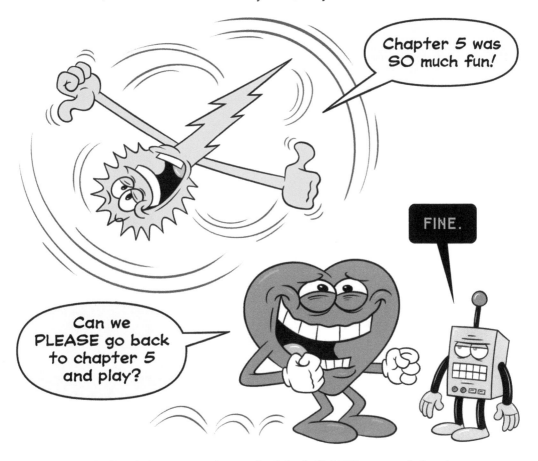

In a nutshell, a left anterior fascicular block (LAFB) causes left axis deviation, while a left posterior fascicular block (LPFB) causes right axis deviation. A block of the LPF is rare. Before making the diagnosis of LPFB it is important to rule out other causes of right axis deviation, including right ventricular hypertrophy and pulmonary disease.

If a fascicular block of the LAF or LPF occurs in isolation, then the ventricle is still depolarized on time by the fibers above the defect and the QRS complex remains fairly narrow. Therefore, the QRS complex in such cases may be of normal duration or only undergo minimal widening of about 0.02 seconds from the its baseline duration. However, fascicular blocks often occur in combination with a bundle branch block, which would result in a wide QRS complex.

LAF vs. LPF: What's the Difference?

A block of the LAF is exceedingly more common than a block of the LPF. This is because the LAF is fragile; it is thin, and only receives a single blood supply from the left anterior descending artery (known as "the widow maker" or LAD).

The LAD also supplies the right bundle branch (RBB). An occlusion of this artery commonly produces a block of the LAF in combination with a right bundle branch block.

In contrast, the LPF is thick and receives a dual blood supply from the LAD and right coronary artery (RCA). A defect of the LPF is very rare.

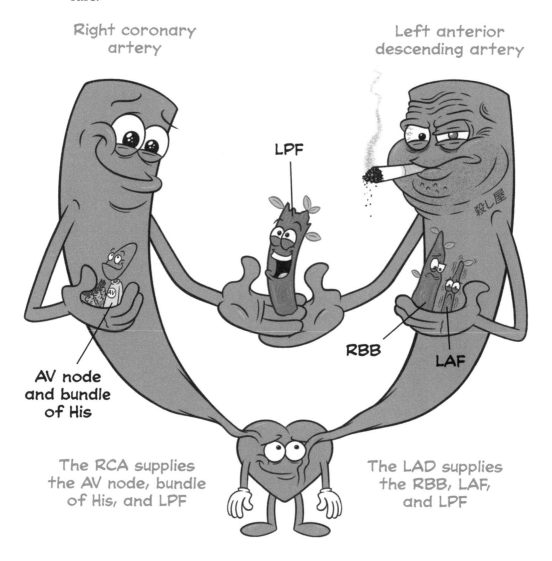

Right coronary artery

Left anterior descending artery

LPF

RBB

LAF

AV node and bundle of His

The RCA supplies the AV node, bundle of His, and LPF

The LAD supplies the RBB, LAF, and LPF

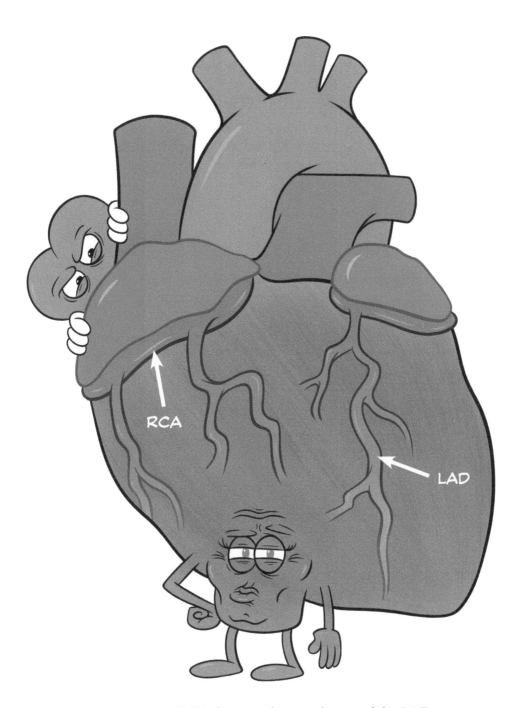

An anterior myocardial infarction due to a lesion of the LAD can cause a LAFB and RBBB.

There are numerous variations in the normal coronary anatomy. This page illustrates an example of a common distribution pattern.

Normal Conduction Through the Fascicles

The left bundle branch gives rise to the LAF and the LPF. The LAF sweeps over the anterosuperior region of the left ventricle, while the LPF sweeps up from an inferoposterior region.

The vectors of electricity follow this spherical path and meet in the middle. Notice that the mean QRS vector is pointing between -30° and +90° on the hexaxial reference system, as we would expect in a normal, healthy heart.

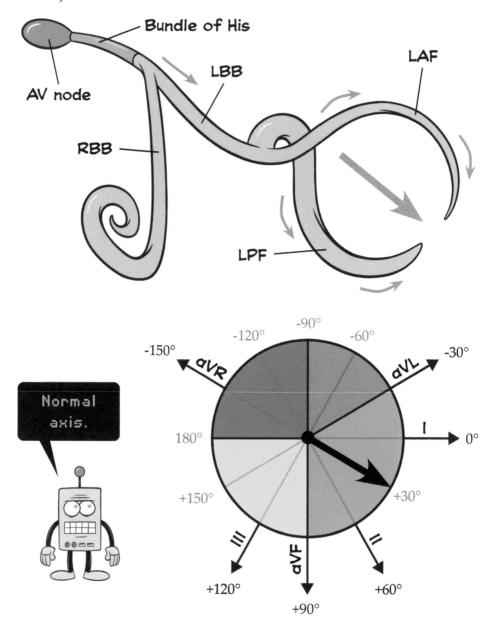

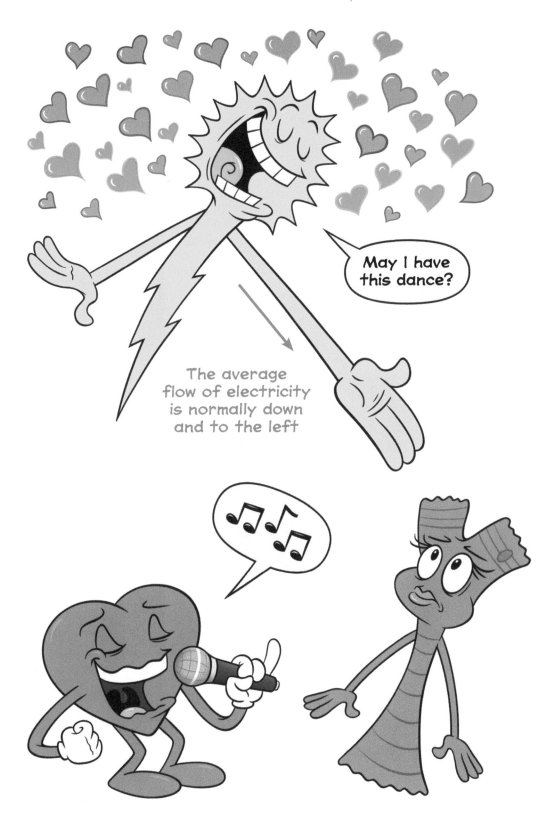

Left Anterior Fascicular Block

If conduction down the LAF is blocked, then the wave of depolarization from the LPF will continue up the circular path unopposed. This electric current depolarizes the area of the left ventricle that the LAF was supposed to supply. Left axis deviation ensues, which is a marker of a diseased heart (especially the left anterior descending artery).

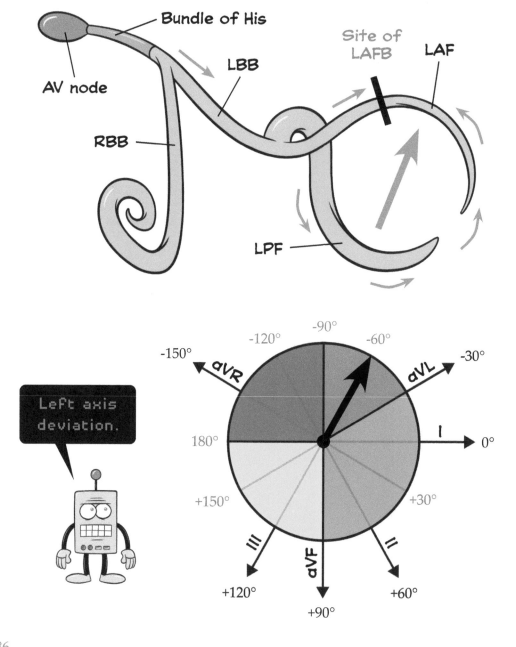

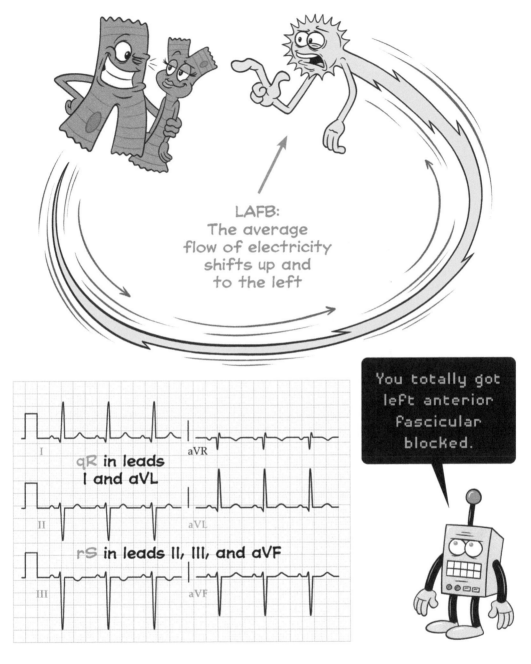

LAFB:
The average
flow of electricity
shifts up and
to the left

qR in leads
I and aVL

I

aVR

II

aVL

rS in leads II, III, and aVF

III

aVF

You totally got left anterior fascicular blocked.

To make the diagnosis of LAFB, there must be an absence of other causes of left axis deviation. Some of the most common causes of left axis deviation can be reviewed on page 95.

LAFB is characterized by left axis deviation, small q waves with tall R waves (qR complexes) in leads I and aVL, and small r waves with deep S waves (rS complexes) in leads II, III, and aVF. The QRS complex may be of normal duration or demonstrate minimal widening.

Left Posterior Fascicular Block

A block to the LPF causes the opposite effects of those described in LAFB. The electric current depolarizes the RBB and sweeps down unopposed from the LAF. This causes the mean QRS vector to shift to right axis deviation. LPFB is very rare, so all other causes of right axis deviation should be ruled out before making the diagnosis of LPFB. Right ventricular hypertrophy is a common cause of right axis deviation.

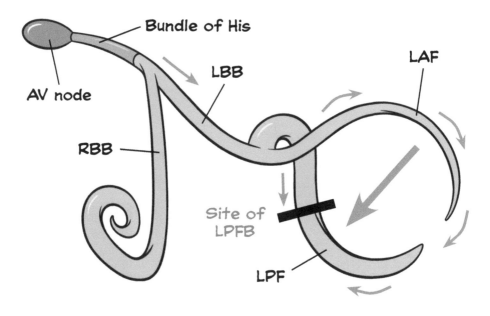

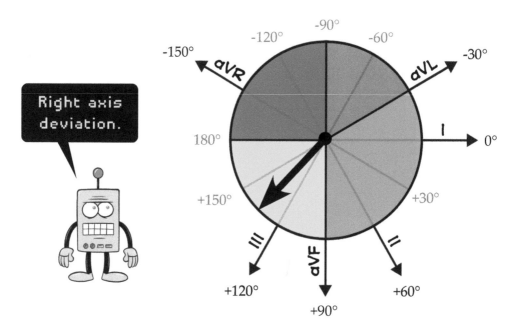

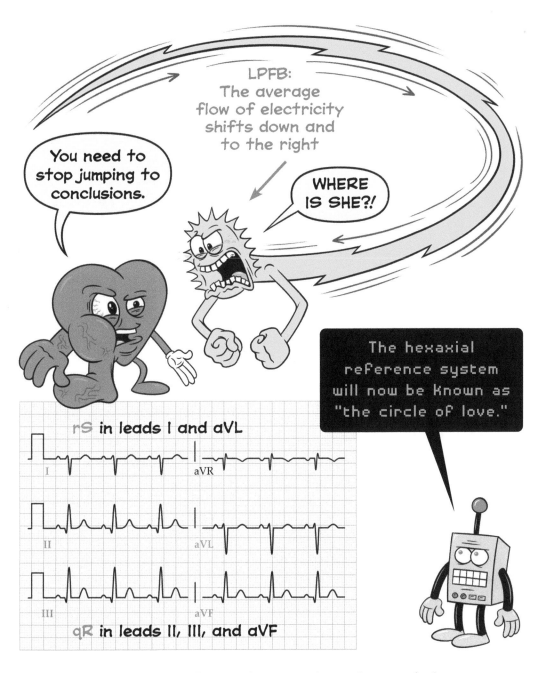

To make the diagnosis of LPFB, there must be an absence of other causes of right axis deviation, such as RVH. Some of the most common causes of right axis deviation can be reviewed on page 95.

LPFB is characterized by right axis deviation, small r waves and deep S (rS complexes) waves in leads I and aVL, and small q waves with tall R waves (qR complexes) in leads II, III, and aVF. The QRS complex may be of normal duration or demonstrate minimal widening.

Bifascicular Block

When a LAFB or LPFB occurs in combination with a RBBB, it is called a bifascicular block. The right bundle branch is also referred to as a separate fascicle, hence the term "bifascicular" block. The most common type of bifascicular block is a RBBB with LAFB because of the shared blood supply from the LAD.

A bifascicular block is worrisome because it means that only one fascicle remains to supply the wave of depolarization to both ventricles. The ECG with bifascicular block will demonstrate a combination of features from the RBBB and either fascicular block.

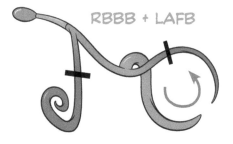

RBBB + LAFB

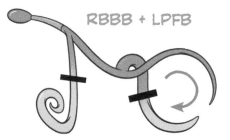

RBBB + LPFB

- QRS complex > 0.12 seconds
- Left axis deviation
- RSR' in leads V1 and V2
- qR complexes in I and aVL
- rS complexes in II, III, and aVF

- QRS complex > 0.12 seconds
- Right axis deviation
- RSR' in leads V1 and V2
- rS complexes in I and aVL
- qR complexes in II, III, and aVF

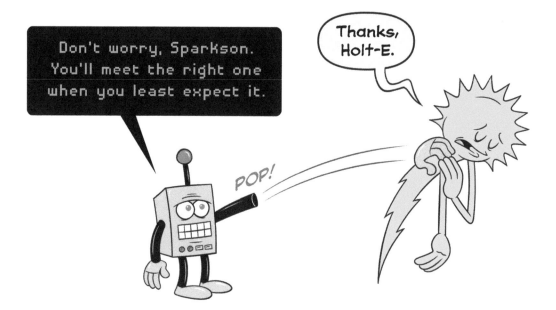

190

Trifascicular Block

A trifascicular block is a conduction block of all three fascicles. It indicates the presence of conduction disease in the right bundle branch in combination with the left anterior and posterior fascicles. A trifascicular block can deteriorate into complete AV block. An ectopic focus would then assume pacing responsibility with a ventricular escape rhythm in order to maintain perfusion.

Complete heart block is considered the terminal stage in the progression of blocks and carries a significant risk of sudden cardiac death. Our goal is to identify bundle branch blocks and fascicular blocks before complete heart block develops. This is important so that patients have the opportunity to seek potentially life-saving treatment such as the insertion of an artificial pacemaker. If a trifascicular block is suspected, the definitive diagnosis is made with electrophysiology studies.

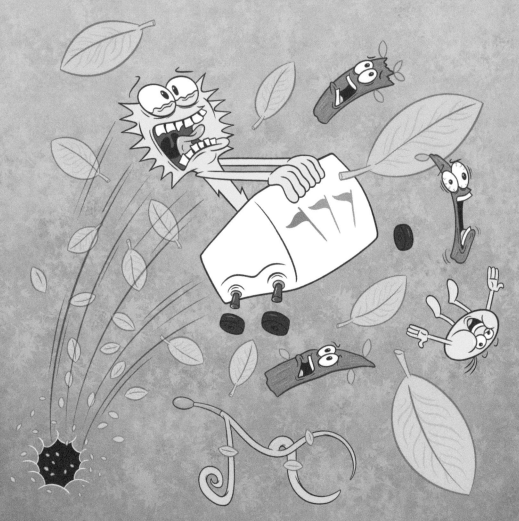

Not all trifascicular blocks are complete. An *incomplete* trifascicular block involves a fixed block in one or two fascicles and an intermittent block in the remaining fascicle(s).

A period of observation is a useful technique to help make this type of diagnosis. Strategies include the use of a Holter monitor or obtaining ECGs for the same patient on different occasions. For example, an ECG may be obtained from a patient that demonstrates a bifascicular block consisting of a RBBB with LAFB. Some time later, an ECG from the same patient demonstrates a RBBB with LPFB. We now have evidence of the alternating failure of the LAF and LPF, and we can infer the presence of disease in all three fascicles.

RBBB + alternating fascicular block

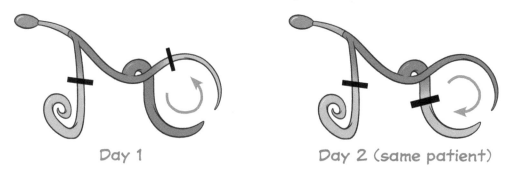

Day 1   Day 2 (same patient)

A fixed RBBB appears in the precordial leads. Serial ECGs demonstrate a variable axis as LAFB alternates with LPFB.

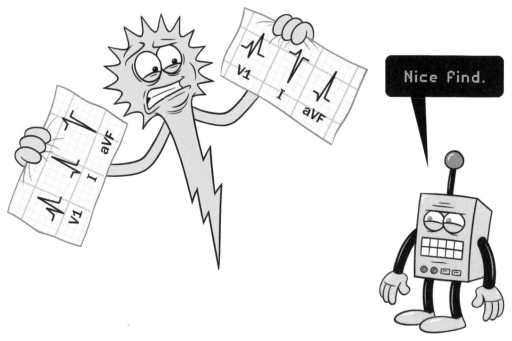

Another type of incomplete trifascicular block consists of a bifascicular block with evidence of delayed conduction in the third fascicle (i.e. first-degree or second-degree AV block pattern).

In this scenario two fascicles maintain a fixed block while the remaining partially diseased fascicle conducts electric impulses very slowly or only conducts some impulses and not others.

If a bifascicular block is diagnosed and the ECG also demonstrates a prolonged PR interval or dropped QRS complexes, the possibility of a diseased third fascicle can be inferred. However, such a pattern could also indicate that the block is occurring at the level of the AV node rather than the third fascicle. The only way to truly localize the origin of the block is with electrophysiology studies.

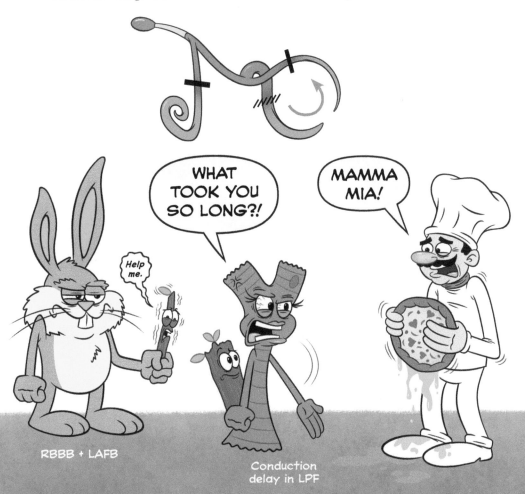

Bifascicular block + first-degree or second-degree block in the remaining fascicle

Pacemakers

Cardiac pacemakers are used to treat arrhythmias that reduce cardiac output or carry a high risk of sudden cardiac death. These sophisticated devices, both temporary and permanent, are able to sense electrical events in the heart and provide an outside source of electrical stimuli when needed. Temporary pacemakers may be inserted in an emergency or serve as a bridge until a permanent pacemaker is placed.

Some of the indications for pacemaker implantation include third-degree AV block, symptomatic second-degree AV block, sick sinus syndrome, symptomatic bradycardia, and for the prevention and termination of recurrent tachyarrhythmias.

The body of a cardiac pacemaker consists of a pulse generator that contains a long-lasting lithium battery. The pulse generator is typically secured in a subcutaneous pocket of tissue below the clavicle.

Lead wires containing an electrode are usually passed transvenously into the right cardiac chambers. Each lead wire contains either one electrode (unipolar lead), or two electrodes (bipolar lead).

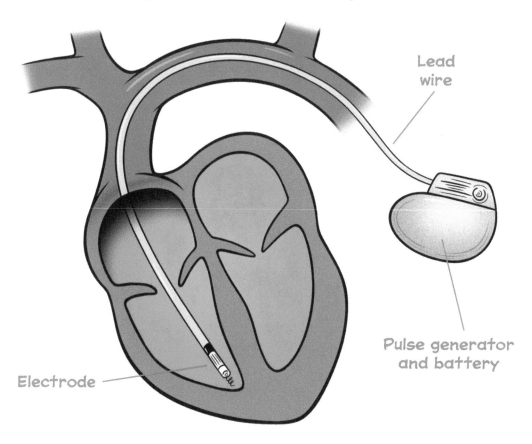

Lead wire

Pulse generator and battery

Electrode

Single chamber pacing systems utilize one lead wire. Dual chamber pacing systems utilize separate lead wires, each placed in the atrium and ventricle. The advantage of dual chamber pacing over ventricular pacing is the ability to mimic normal cardiac behavior by maintaining AV synchrony.

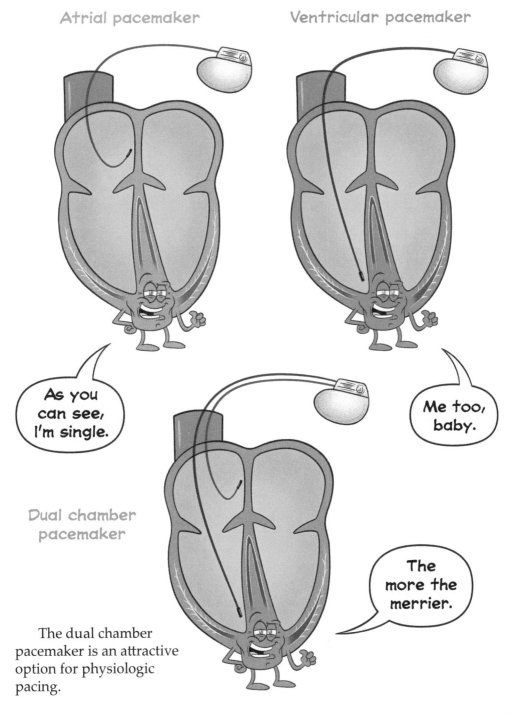

Atrial pacemaker

Ventricular pacemaker

As you can see, I'm single.

Me too, baby.

Dual chamber pacemaker

The more the merrier.

The dual chamber pacemaker is an attractive option for physiologic pacing.

The depolarization of the atria or ventricles in response to a pacing stimulus is called *capture*. The electrodes inside the heart are able to deliver electric impulses to the myocardium to initiate waves depolarization.

The pacemaker's regular pacing activity is recorded as narrow spikes on the ECG. Sometimes the spikes are very small and difficult to see. In those cases a thorough history and physical examination should reveal whether or not an artificial pacemaker is present.

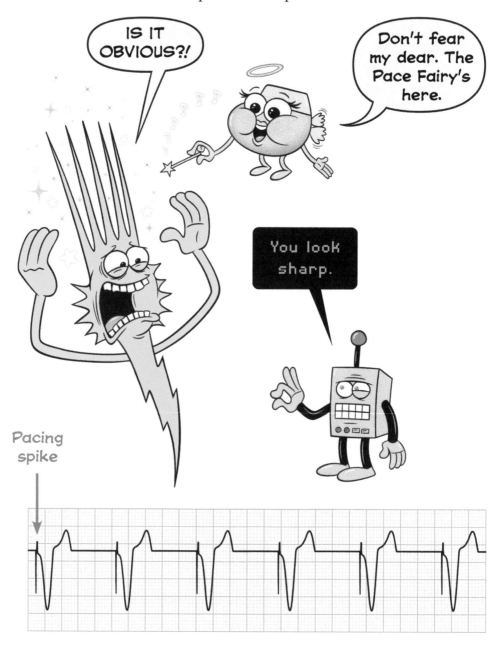

Pacemaker Nomenclature

A five-letter coding system has been developed to identify the functions of a permanent pacemaker. The first three positions of the code are most commonly used. When a code only utilizes the first three or four positions, it can be assumed that the remaining positions are absent.

- **Position I:** The first position designates the chamber(s) being paced.

  A: atrium
  V: ventricle
  D: dual (atrium and ventricle)
  O: none

- **Position II:** The second position refers to the chamber(s) in which the pacemaker senses cardiac electrical activity.

  A: atrium
  V: ventricle
  D: dual (atrium and ventricle)
  O: none

- **Position III:** The third position indicates how the pacemaker responds to sensed cardiac electrical activity.

  I: sensed activity inhibits pacing
  T: sensed activity triggers pacing
  D: dual modes of response (pacing can be triggered and inhibited)
  O: none (no pacemaker response to electrical activity)

- **Position IV:** The fourth position indicates the pacemaker's ability or inability for rate modulation. The presence of this rate-adaptive mechanism indicates the pacemaker is equipped with a sensor that can adjust its programmed pacing rate in response to physiological activity.

  R: rate modulation present
  O: none (rate modulation absent)

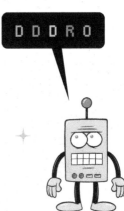

- **Position V:** The fifth position refers to the presence of multisite pacing in the atrium, ventricle, or both.

  A: atrium
  V: ventricle
  D: dual (atrial and ventricular multisite pacing)
  O: none

A pacemaker provides 100 percent capture if the heart depends entirely on the device for pacing. However, many pacemakers have a *demand* mode in which the device only delivers an electric impulse if the heart's intrinsic rate dips below a preset level. In this respect, the pacemaker is overdrive-suppressed when the heart is depolarizing within normal limits, but is able to escape to provide intermittent capture when it does not sense intrinsic activity from the heart.

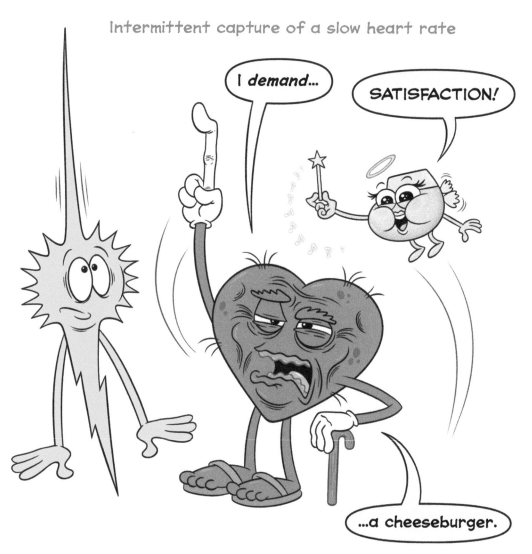

Intermittent capture of a slow heart rate

On the other hand, tachyarrhythmias can also develop in the presence of a pacemaker. The device can respond to these cases if it has been programmed to sense an increase in the intrinsic heart rate. It would then speed up its own rate to overdrive-suppress the heart and assume pacing control. Once this is achieved, the pacemaker can slow the heart to a desired rate, thereby terminating the tachyarrhythmia.

Pacemaker Modes

The ideal pacing mode should be selected depending on the patient's clinical condition and underlying arrhythmia. Some examples of pacing modes are AAI, VVI, and DDD.

AAI, also known as atrial demand pacing, is a single chamber pacing system that paces the atrium and senses atrial impulses. When intrinsic atrial activity with a rate greater than a predetermined level is sensed, pacing will be inhibited and the pacemaker resets itself. If the pacemaker does not sense the critical electric activity from the atrium, then it will assume pacing responsibility.

Atrial demand pacing is utilized in patients that have symptomatic sinus node dysfunction with a normally functioning AV node. This mode is used infrequently because it does not offer protection from ventricular bradyarrhythmias caused by to AV block.

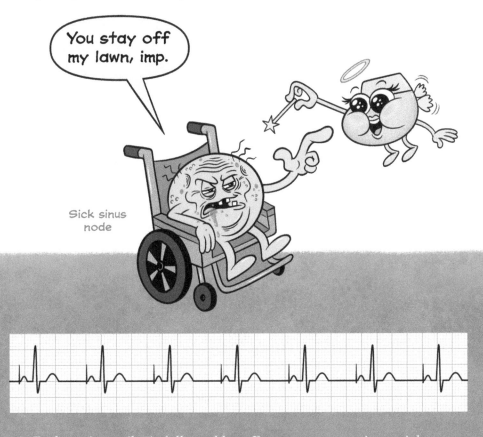

Each pacing spike is followed by a P wave, representing atrial depolarization. An intact AV node allows transmission to the ventricles.

U U I, also known as ventricular demand pacing, is a single chamber pacing system that paces the ventricle and senses ventricular impulses. It functions similar to the AAI mode. The VVI pacemaker generates an impulse whenever the heart's intrinsic ventricular rate falls below the programmed level. If intrinsic ventricular impulses are sensed within normal limits, then pacing will be inhibited. Ventricular demand pacing is useful in the setting of chronic atrial fibrillation with a slow ventricular response or complete AV block.

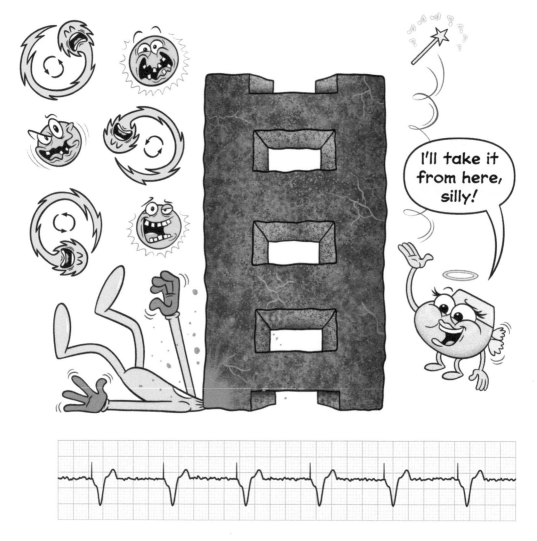

I'll take it from here, silly!

The VVI pacemaker produces a spike followed by a wide QRS complex. The electrode is usually placed in the right ventricular apex, causing a wave of depolarization that generally spreads through the heart in a right-to-left direction. This creates a LBBB pattern on the ECG.

Single chamber ventricular pacing is associated with a complication known as *pacemaker syndrome*. This condition describes a decrease in cardiac output that develops when the timing of contractions between the atria and the ventricles are unsynchronized. Loss of AV synchrony is correlated with heart failure and may lead to symptoms including fatigue, shortness of breath, and lightheadedness. Pacemaker syndrome can be avoided by inserting a pacing system that is able to maintain AV synchrony such as a dual chamber pacemaker.

D D D is a dual chamber pacing system consisting of atrial and ventricular leads that are both capable of pacing and sensing. This is a common and versatile pacing mode that automatically adjusts to the heart's intrinsic electrical activity and is designed to ensure AV synchrony. The DDD pacemaker is commonly used in cases of SA node dysfunction (e.g., sick sinus syndrome) and AV block.

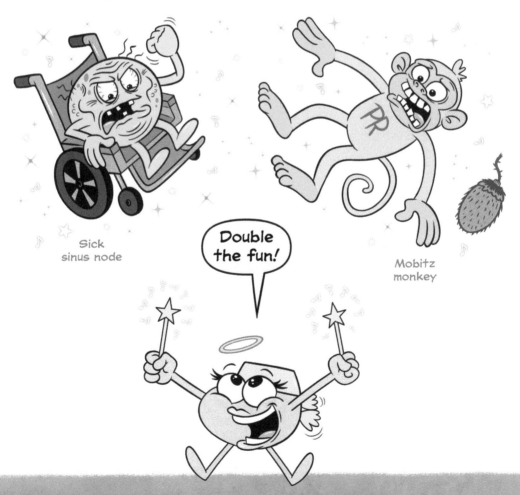

Sick sinus node

Double the fun!

Mobitz monkey

A normally functioning DDD pacemaker is associated with four different rhythms depending on the heart's intrinsic activity:

Complete inhibition

The pacemaker is completely inhibited as it senses intrinsic impulses from the atria and ventricles at a rate within normal programmed limits. Pacing spikes are absent from the tracing.

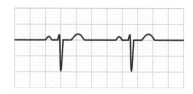

Atrial pacing with conduction

Atrial pacing occurs when the intrinsic atrial rate falls below the programmed limit. An intact AV node conducts the paced impulse to the ventricles which results in a native QRS complex.

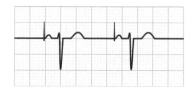

Atrial sensing, ventricular pacing

The pacemaker senses a native atrial impulse that inhibits the device from firing. However, the impulse fails to conduct to the ventricles which results in a paced QRS complex.

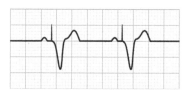

AV sequential pacing

Coordinated atrial and ventricular pacing occurs as conduction depends entirely on the pacemaker. This rhythm may be seen, for example, in the setting of sinus bradycardia with AV block.

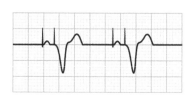

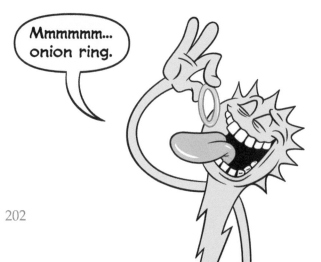

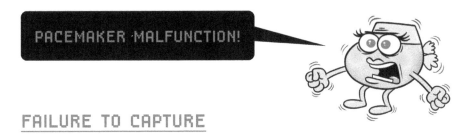

PACEMAKER MALFUNCTION!

FAILURE TO CAPTURE

When a pacemaker fails to depolarize a heart that is physiologically capable of being stimulated, it is termed failure to capture. The pacemaker is unsuccessful at stimulating a contraction, which is reflected on the ECG as a pacing spike without a P wave or QRS complex response.

The causes of failure to capture include lead wire displacement, lead wire fracture, inflammation and fibrosis at the site of the electrode, or metabolic disturbances (e.g. hyperkalemia, acidosis and alkalosis). It can also be caused by medications that increase the pacing threshold such as flecainide and propafenone (class IC drugs).

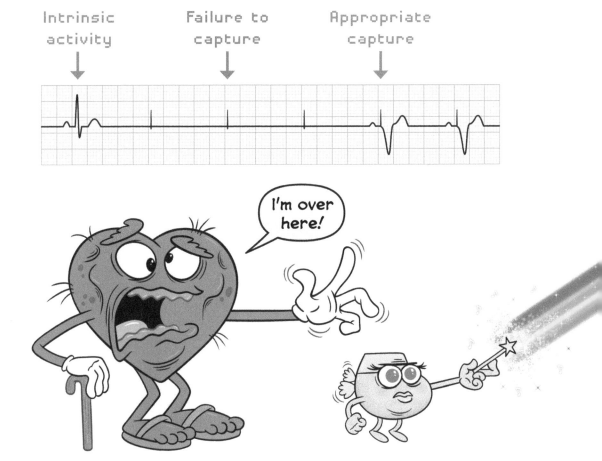

FAILURE TO PACE

Failure to pace is recognized as the absence of pacing spikes when there is an indication for pacing. Causes include battery depletion, lead wire displacement, lead wire fracture, and oversensing.

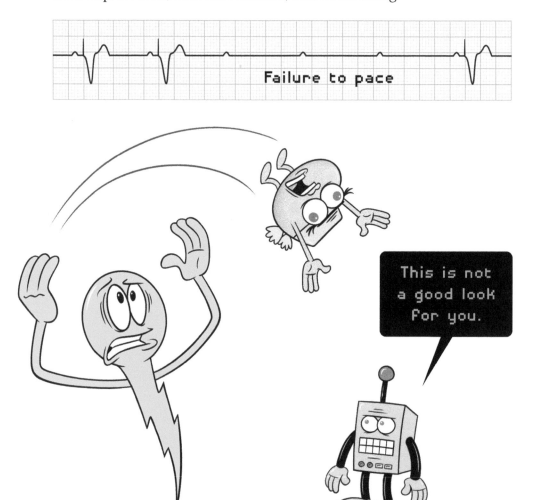

OVERSENSING

Oversensing occurs when the pacemaker misinterprets outside electrical stimuli to be intrinsic cardiac activity and withholds pacing. Failure to pace occurs because the pacemaker is too sensitive to the surrounding environment. Sources of potential interference include MRI, radiation therapy, electrocautery, arc welding, transcutaneous electrical nerve stimulation (TENS), and extracorporeal shock wave lithotripsy.

UNDERSENSING

Undersensing occurs when the pacemaker fails to detect intrinsic electrical activity and fires inappropriately. Spikes might appear in the middle or after native P waves and QRS complexes. These spikes are especially dangerous because if one them falls on a T wave it could set off a malignant ventricular arrhythmia (R on T phenomenon). Undersensing is caused by many of the same mechanical and physiologic disturbances that cause failure to capture.

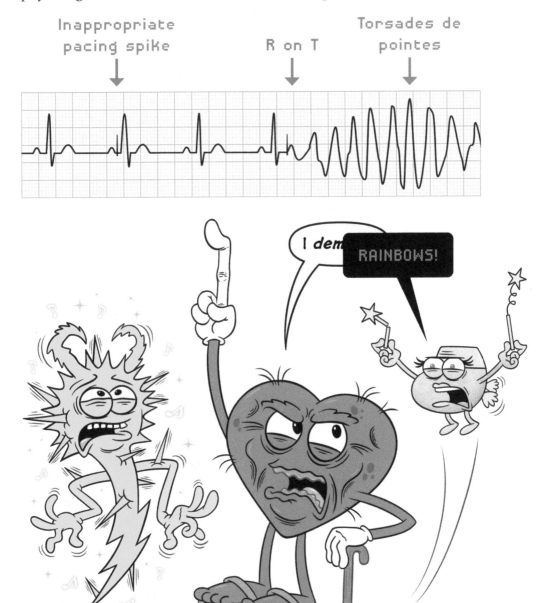

Inappropriate pacing spike

R on T

Torsades de pointes

I dem RAINBOWS!

Biventricular Pacemaker

Biventricular pacing is also known as cardiac resynchronization therapy (CRT). It is used in the management of heart failure with ventricular dyssynchrony, which may cause a prolonged QRS complex. CRT reduces symptoms and improves overall quality of life in patients with heart failure. Most candidates for CRT also meet the criteria for ICD placement and receive a combined device.

A biventricular pacemaker utilizes an additional lead wire placed in the coronary sinus to reach the left ventricular wall. Lead wires are also placed in the right ventricle and usually the right atrium. This configuration allows the pacemaker to capture the left and right ventricles simultaneously and appropriately synchronize ventricular contractions.

Indications

- QRS duration ≥ 0.15 seconds
- Left ventricular ejection fraction ≤ 35 percent
- Symptomatic heart failure despite optimal medical therapy
- New York Heart Association (NYHA) class II, III, or IV heart failure

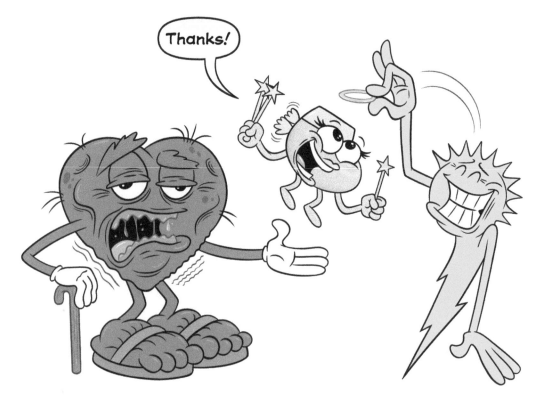

Sparkson's Summary: Chapter 8

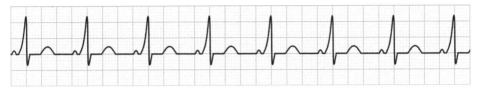

Wolff-Parkinson White syndrome: short PR interval, wide QRS complex, and delta wave

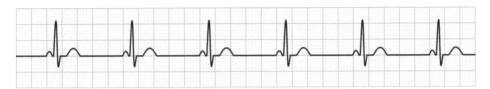

Lown-Ganong-Levine syndrome: short PR interval, narrow QRS complex

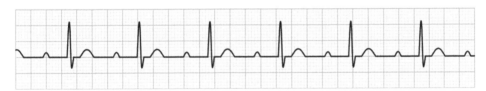

First-degree AV block: PR interval longer than 0.2 seconds, consistently long each cycle

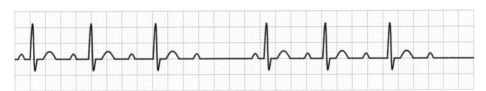

Mobitz type I AV block: progressive prolongation of the PR interval until a QRS complex is dropped

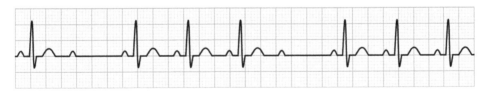

Mobitz type II AV block: the PR interval does not lengthen before or after the dropped QRS complex

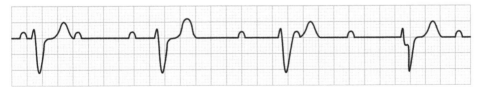

Third-degree (complete heart block): P waves and QRS complexes are completely independent

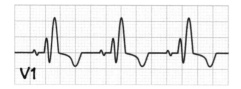 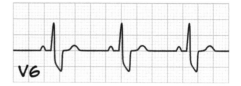

RBBB: wide QRS complex, RSR' pattern in lead V1 and wide, slurred S waves in lead V6

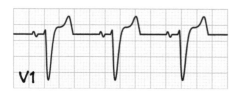 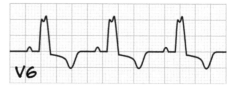

LBBB: broad, deep S waves in lead V1 and wide, notched (or slurred) R waves in lead V6

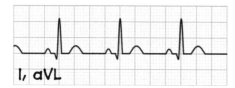 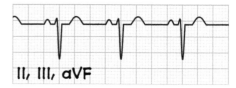

LAFB: left axis deviation, qR in leads I and aVL, rS in leads II, III, and aVF

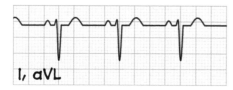 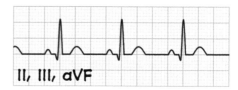

LPFB: right axis deviation, rS in leads I and aVL, qR in leads II, III, and aVF

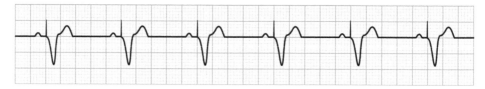

Atrial-sensed, ventricular paced rhythm

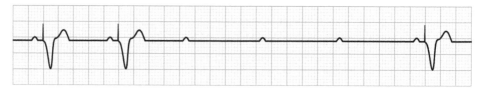

Failure to pace

CHAPTER 9

MYOCARDIAL INFARCTION (AND FRIENDS)

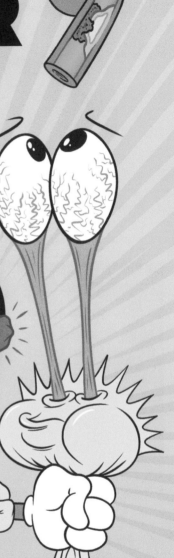

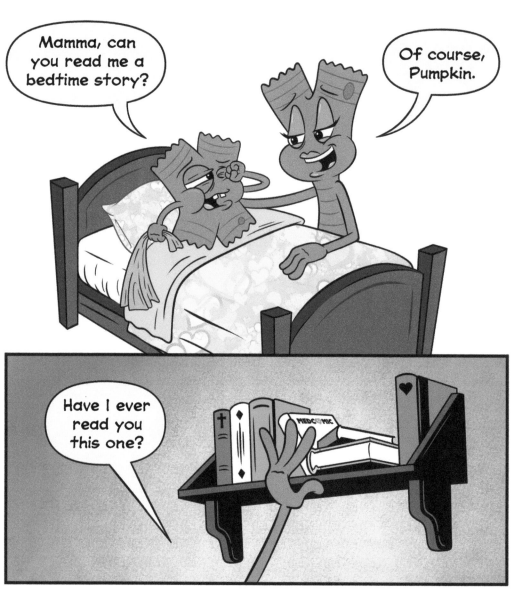

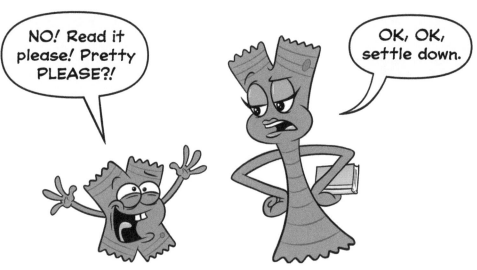

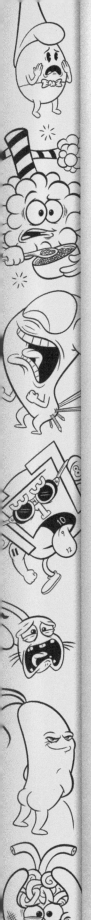

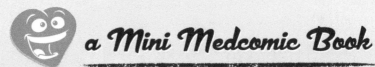
a Mini Medcomic Book

The lad named "Lad"

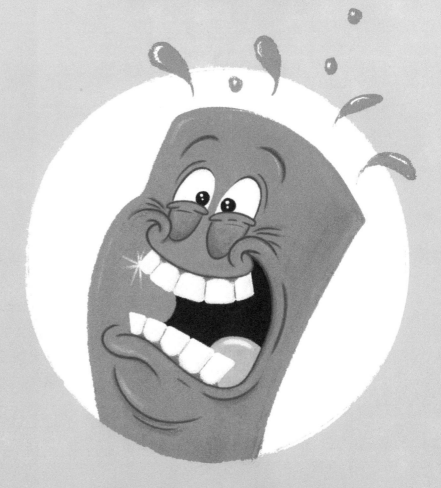

By Jorge Muniz

There once was a lad named "Lad",
jolly and happy and glad.
He ate what he wanted
to excess and flaunted
how great of a life he had.

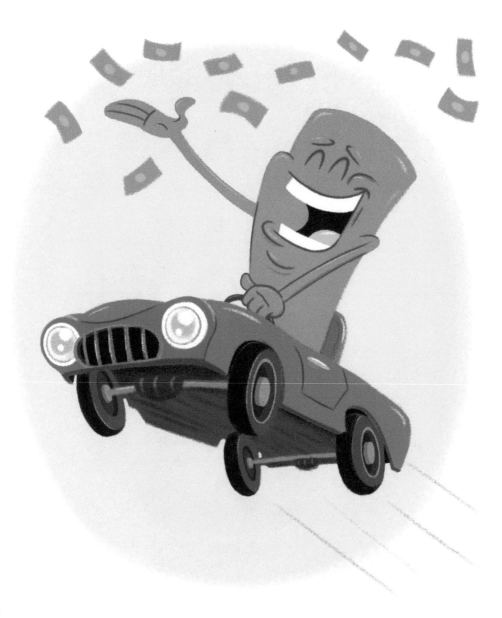

Lad loved onion rings and bread
with extra butter to spread.
"Glazed donuts for dessert!
Three or four wouldn't hurt,"
is what the lad always said.

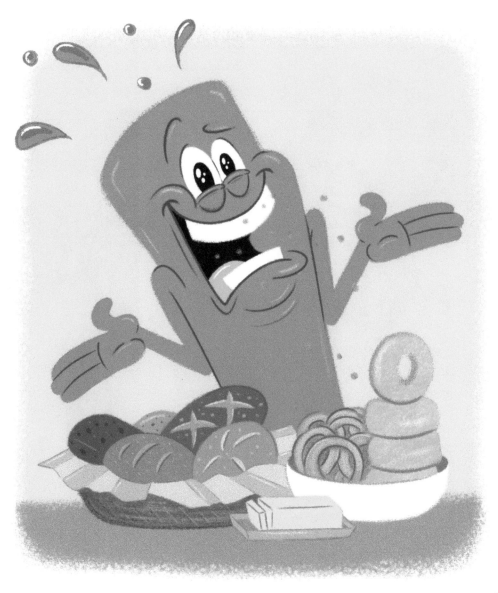

Lad's blood sugar quickly rose.

Pins and needles struck his toes.

He despised a long jog,

was as still as a log,

watching his favorite shows.

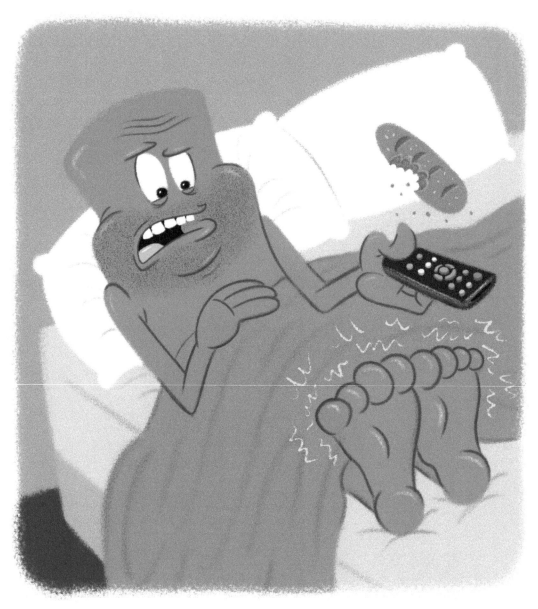

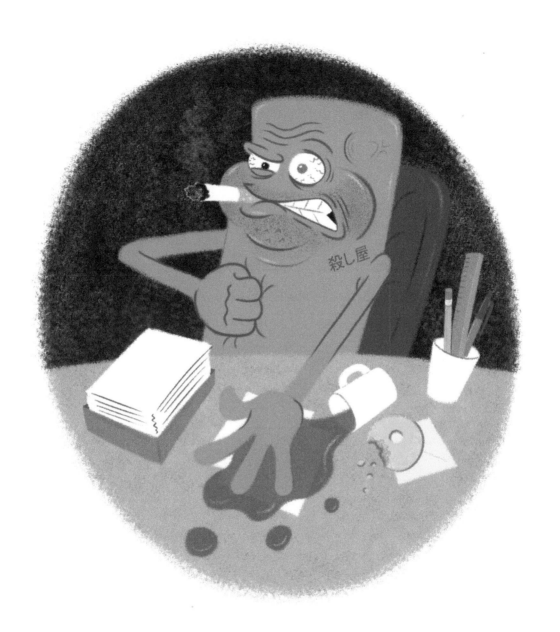

Long work hours got Lad stressed.

He smoked and never got rest.

His dad passed like a breeze

from cardiac disease

and Lad felt pain in his chest.

Lad's tires screeched on pavement!
Straight to the ED he went.
Surely he'll give his health
the importance of wealth
after receiving a stent?

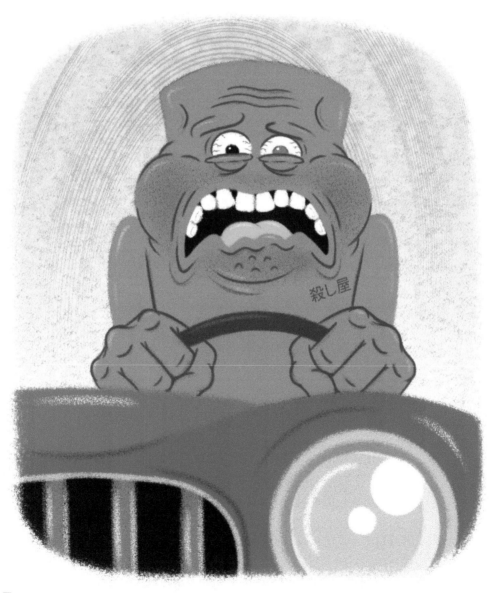

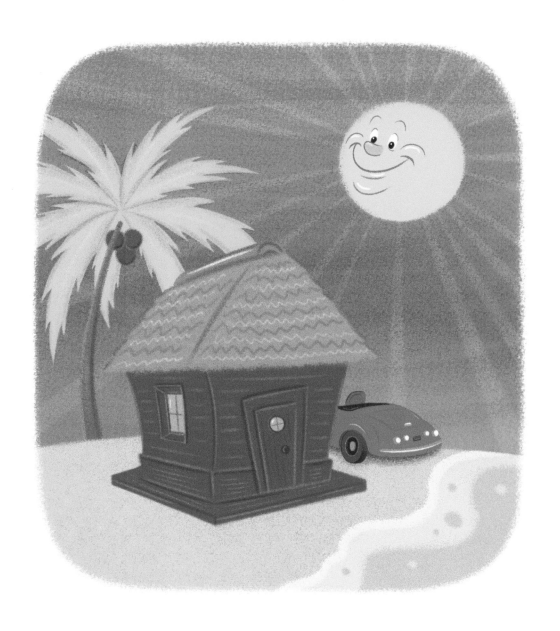

But he stubbornly denied

his hypertension flood tide.

Without medication,

Lad went on vacation,

choked on a blood clot and died.

6

ISBN 978-0-9966513-1-8

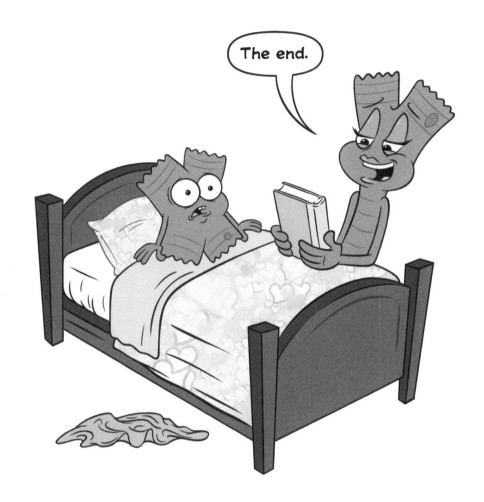

Coronary Thrombosis

The most common cause of myocardial infarction (MI) is coronary thrombosis. A coronary artery may narrow over time as a result of atherosclerotic plaque buildup beneath the intimal lining of the vessel. This plaque can become unstable and rupture, leading to the formation of an acute thrombus and subsequent occlusion of the artery.

All myocardial cells need oxygen to survive. The region of the myocardium supplied by an occluded artery loses its blood supply, creating an imbalance in myocardial oxygen supply and demand. Unless circulation and oxygenation is restored, the myocardial cells undergo the pathologic processes of ischemia, injury, and infarction.

Risk factors for coronary artery disease include a high fat, high carbohydrate diet, diabetes, obesity, a sedentary lifestyle, stress, smoking, a family history of heart disease, and hypertension. Can you find all of these in "The Lad Named Lad"?

Ischemia, Injury, and Infarction

Damage to myocardial cells can develop through any process that increases the demand for oxygen or that results in a decreased blood supply. Coronary thrombosis due to plaque rupture is the most common cause, but examples of less common etiologies include coronary artery vasospasm, coronary artery dissection, and stent thrombosis.

Occlusion of a vessel initiates three stages along a continuum: myocardial ischemia, injury, and infarction.

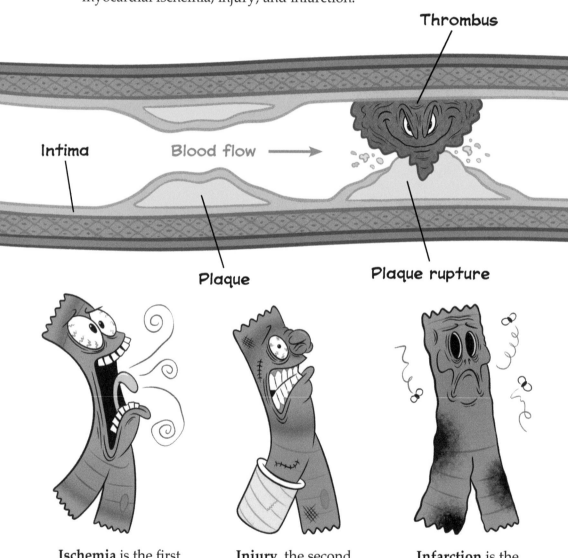

Ischemia is the first stage that occurs when myocardial cells are gasping for oxygen.

Injury, the second stage, represents cell damage due to prolonged ischemia.

Infarction is the third stage and occurs with irreversible myocardial cell death.

Layers of the Heart

The heart is enclosed in a double-layered sac called the pericardium. The outer layer is named the fibrous pericardium and the inner layer is named the serous pericardium. The serous pericardium is distinguished further by an outer parietal layer and an inner visceral layer which are continuous with each other. The pericardial cavity is located between them, which contains the pericardial fluid that lubricates the heart.

The heart wall has three main tissue layers. The heart's outermost layer is called the epicardium, which is another name for the visceral layer of the serous pericardium. The main coronary arteries lie on the epicardial surface of the heart. They supply oxygen and nutrients to this layer before entering the middle layer of the heart, known as the myocardium.

The myocardium is a thick, muscular layer which consists of the cardiomyocytes responsible for the pumping action of the heart. The myocardium is subdivided into two layers. The outermost half of the myocardium is called the subepicardium. The innermost half is called the subendocardium. **The subendocardium is at the greatest risk for ischemia and infarction because this layer receives blood from the most distal branches of the coronary arteries and has a high demand for oxygen.**

The heart's innermost layer is called the endocardium. It's made up of a thin layer of epithelial tissue and connective tissue that lines the heart's chambers and valves.

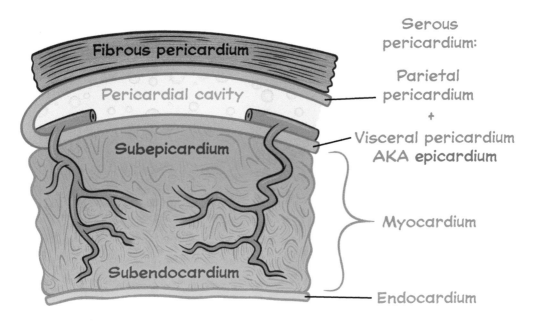

Acute Coronary Syndrome

Acute coronary syndrome (ACS) is an umbrella term that describes a group of diseases caused by ischemia of the myocardium. The degree of blockage and the time that the affected vessel remains obstructed determines the severity of disease progression.

ACS consists of three main conditions: unstable *angina (UA), non-ST-elevation myocardial infarction (NSTEMI), and ST-elevation myocardial infarction (STEMI). UA and NSTEMI have also been grouped together under the designation of non-ST-elevation ACS (NSTE-ACS).

Unstable angina is usually caused by partial or intermittent coronary obstruction. It can progress to myocardial infarction, which involves total coronary obstruction.

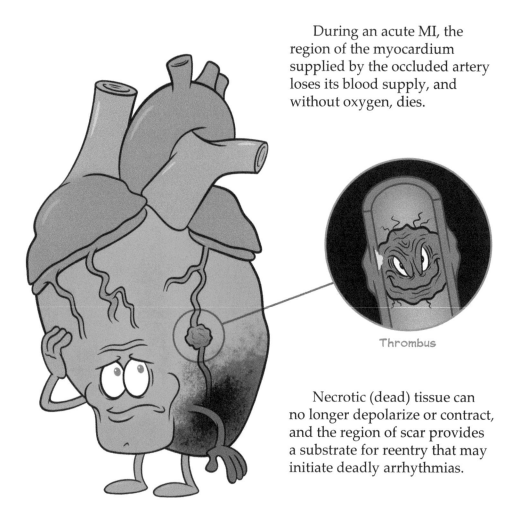

During an acute MI, the region of the myocardium supplied by the occluded artery loses its blood supply, and without oxygen, dies.

Thrombus

Necrotic (dead) tissue can no longer depolarize or contract, and the region of scar provides a substrate for reentry that may initiate deadly arrhythmias.

*Angina is the characteristic chest pain associated with coronary artery disease.

The clinical presentation of ACS may include chest pain or chest pressure, pain from the chest that radiates to the jaw or left arm, shortness of breath, diaphoresis, and nausea. In many clinical scenarios ACS will not present according to this "classic" description. Diabetics, females, and elderly patients are more likely to experience atypical chest pain compared to other patient populations in the setting of ACS .

The occlusion of a coronary artery is a dynamic process. A partial or intermittent occlusion may progress into a complete blockage, which usually manifests on the ECG as a STEMI. Evolutionary ECG changes can be captured by obtaining serial ECGs on a patient. NSTEMI and UA are differentiated from one another by obtaining biomarkers such as troponins, which are typically absent in UA.

Cardiac biomarkers are useful for the diagnosis and prognosis of myocardial infarction. Myoglobin lacks specificity, rises in 1 to 4 hours, and returns to normal within 24 hours. Creatine kinase (CK-MB) is the classic biomarker of an acute MI. It's found primarily in cardiac muscle, and in small amounts in skeletal muscle and the brain. CK-MB rises in 4 to 12 hours and returns to normal within 36 to 48 hours. Cardiac troponins are the preferred biomarkers for the diagnosis of an acute MI. They are the most sensitive and specific serologic test. Troponins rise in 4 to 12 hours and may remain elevated for up to two weeks.

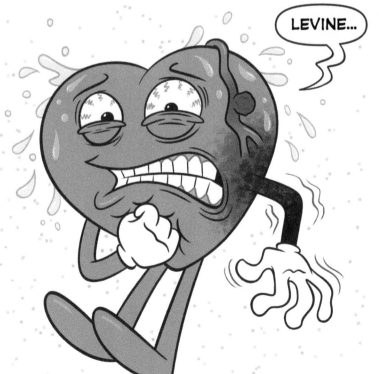

LEVINE...

Troponins

- Most sensitive and specific
- Rise in 4-12 hours
- May remain elevated for up to two weeks

CK-MB

- Rises in 4-12 hours
- Returns to normal within 36-48 hours

Myoglobin

- Lacks specificity
- Rises in 1-4 hours
- Returns to normal within 24 hours

ECG Manifestations of ACS

An ECG should be obtained immediately in the setting of new-onset chest pain suspicious for ACS. This is performed to see if there are any ECG changes indicating ischemia or infarction. Most MIs manifest on the ECG with characteristic changes that lead to the correct diagnosis.

These ECG findings include ST depression or elevation, T wave inversion, pathologic Q waves, new axis deviation, poor R wave progression, and various types of conduction blocks (e.g. bundle branch block or AV block). Unstable angina and NSTEMI may or may not manifest with ST depression and T wave inversion. The ECG in these two syndromes could even be normal.

It is always helpful to obtain a prior ECG from the patient's records to have a baseline ECG to compare to. If cardiac biomarkers are positive, the ECG can help determine the severity of the MI. The most common way of categorizing an MI is according to elevation of the T segment (i.e. STEMI vs. NSTEMI).

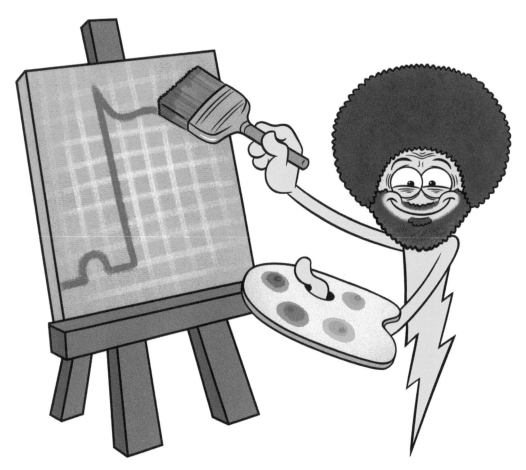

Stress Testing

ECG monitoring is utilized during a stress test, which is a non-invasive method of detecting coronary artery disease (CAD). It is also used for risk stratification and monitoring of known CAD.

Stress testing induces an episode of increased oxygen demand in order to identify evidence of cardiac ischemia on the ECG. Blood flow to the heart is increased with the use of physical exercise or stimulated chemically with medications. Exercise stress testing is only reliable in patients that do not have baseline ECG abnormalities at rest which would interfere with interpretation of the results.

Pharmacologic stress testing is usually reserved for patients that cannot tolerate physical exercise due to conditions such as arthritis, claudication, or pulmonary disease, among many others. A myocardial perfusion scan provides nuclear images of the heart under stress and at rest, which are then compared for evidence of defects or ischemia.

A treadmill or stationary bicycle is ordinarily used for exercise stress testing. The workload increases incrementally until the patient reaches a predetermined endpoint established by protocol. The test would end before the predetermined endpoint if the patient developed signs or symptoms indicative of cardiac disease. ST segment deviation is the most important ECG change indicative of CAD during a stress test. ST segment depression is a sign of myocardial ischemia.

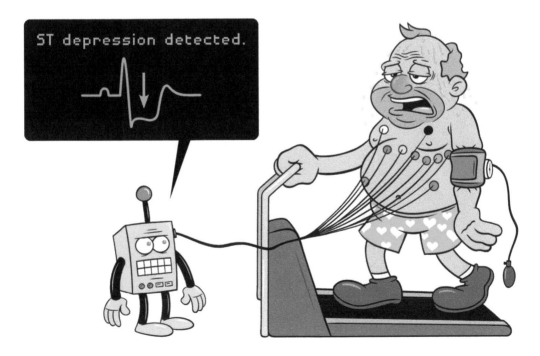

Measuring ST Segment Deviation

The J point is the junction between the end of the S wave and the beginning of the ST segment. ST elevation or depression is calculated by measuring deviation of the J point relative to the PR segment. In other words, the PR segment is the reference line to which elevation or depression of the J point is compared. ST segment elevation greater than 1 mm or ST depression greater than 0.5 mm is considered abnormal.

A STEMI is diagnosed by the presence of new ST segment elevation in two or more contiguous leads, detailed by the following criteria:

- Greater than 1 mm of ST elevation in leads other than V2 and V3
- For leads V2 and V3, the following cut-points apply:
  ≥ 2 mm in men ≥ 40 years old, ≥ 2.5 mm in men < 40 years old, or ≥ 1.5 mm in women

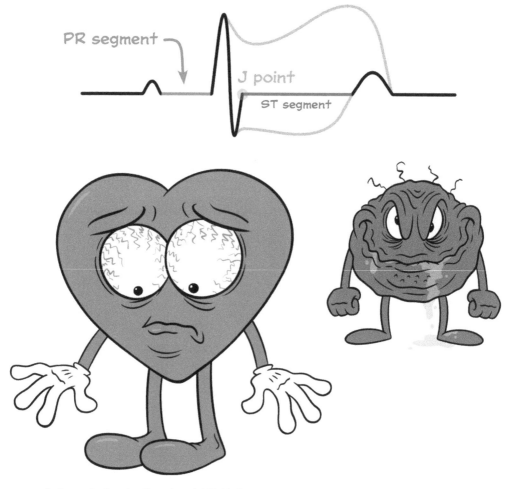

Author note: there's a thrombus *right behind you.*

ECG Changes Following an Acute MI

The ECG can help us determine the approximate age of an infarct. The ECG of a heart undergoing infarction evolves over minutes, hours, days, weeks, and even years following an acute occlusion.

There are three main components of the ECG that evolve after the onset of an acute MI. Changes occur to the T waves, ST segment, and QRS complex due to the effects of ischemia, injury, and infarction.

Hyperacute T waves appear immediately after an occlusion. The T waves become very tall, narrow, and represent the earliest stage of an infarct in progress. These peaked T waves frequently go unobserved because of their transient nature.

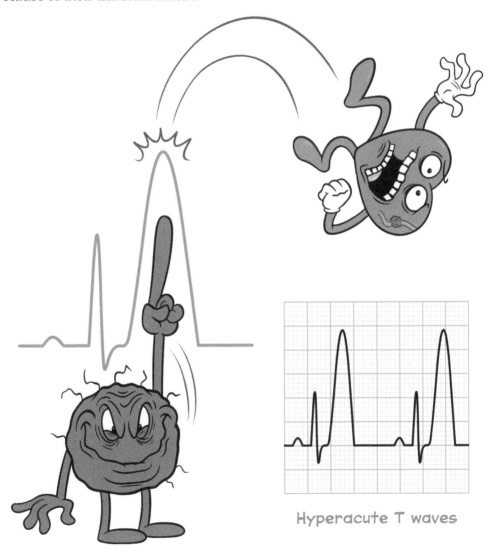

Hyperacute T waves

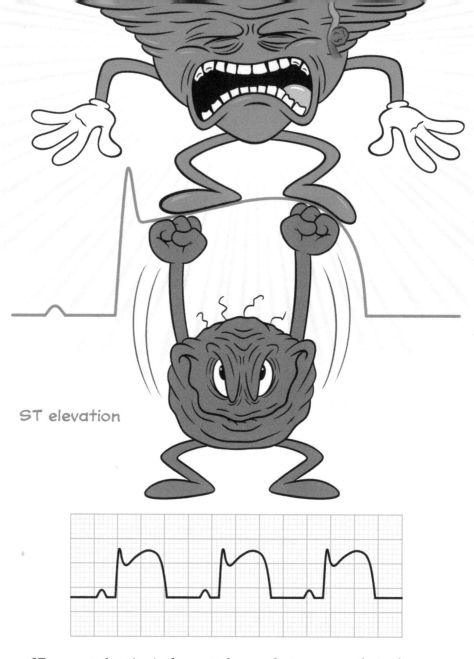

ST elevation

ST segment elevation is the next change that occurs early in the progression of an acute MI. It is a sign of myocardial cell injury beyond ischemia. The morphology of ST segment elevation evolves rapidly with characteristic patterns that can be followed with serial ECGs. As the height of the ST segment increases it tends to become convex, like a frown.

ST segment elevation persists anywhere from a few hours to several days and then returns to baseline. ST elevation that persists for more than two weeks is indicative of the formation of a *ventricular aneurysm*. This is a complication of infarction in which the necrotic ventricular wall becomes thin and bulges. ST elevation can also be caused by a number of other conditions which will be discussed later in this chapter.

Reciprocal changes refer to mirror image ECG patterns that occur in leads "opposite" from the site of an acute MI. They appear because the surface electrodes are viewing the same electrical activity from a different angle. Reciprocal changes usually manifest in the form of ST segment depression in leads distant from the site of infarction.

For example, an acute STEMI of the inferior heart wall would produce ST elevation in leads II, III, and aVF. Reciprocal changes in the form of ST depression may be seen simultaneously in leads I and aVL.

Reciprocal changes do not always occur, but their presence on the ECG is a strong indicator of acute infarction.

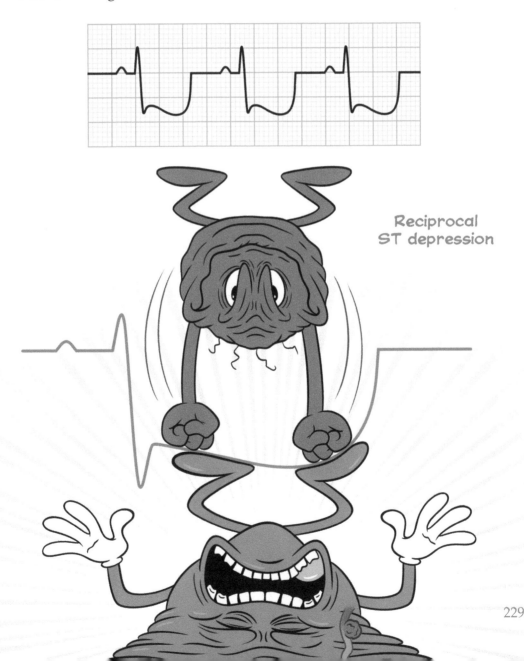

Reciprocal
ST depression

T wave inversion generally occurs after deviation of the ST segment and indicates myocardial ischemia. The T wave inversion is characteristically deep and symmetrical. Signs of ischemia on the ECG can be reversed if blood flow is restored. It is also possible for T wave inversions to remain on the ECG for months or persist indefinitely.

T wave inversion is a nonspecific finding in isolation. It can be found in numerous other conditions including ventricular hypertrophy and bundle branch block. However, the symmetrical nature of the ischemic T wave is a clue that it is a manifestation of ACS. In most other conditions, the inverted T wave is associated with a downsloping ST segment that returns sharply to baseline.

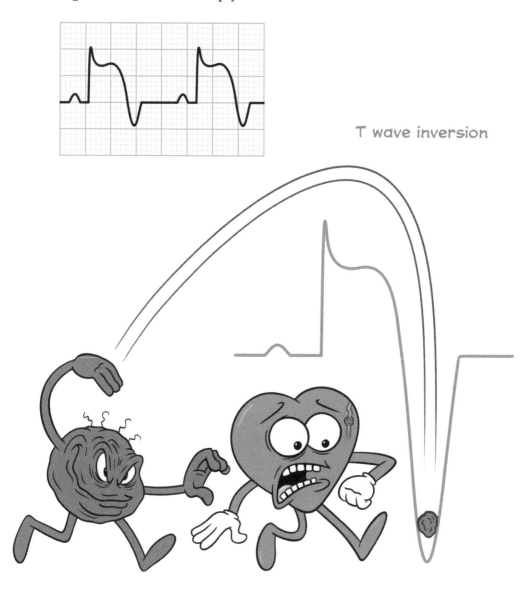

T wave inversion

The final ECG change that may occur from acute infarction is the development of *pathologic Q waves* (also known as *significant Q waves*). They appear within several hours after the onset of an acute MI. Pathologic Q waves indicate myocardial necrosis and they usually persist on the ECG as permanent signs of a prior MI. However, pathologic Q waves may get smaller with time or even disappear.

To be considered pathologic, the Q wave should be greater than 0.04 seconds (one small box) in duration or have an amplitude greater than one-fourth of the R wave in the same lead. Duration is more important than amplitude in the assessment of Q waves for evidence of pathology.

It is normal for lead aVR to contain a deep Q wave because it is oriented to record activity from the right upper side of the heart.

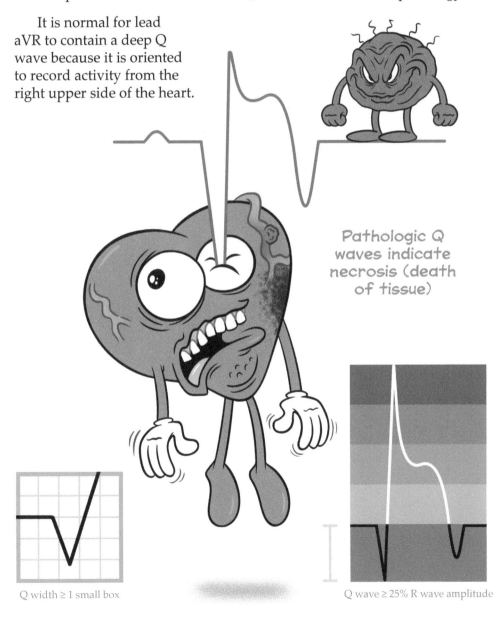

Pathologic Q waves indicate necrosis (death of tissue)

Q width ≥ 1 small box

Q wave ≥ 25% R wave amplitude

Septal Q Waves

Small septal Q waves are a normal finding in the left lateral leads (I, aVL, V5, and V6) and inferior leads (II, III, and aVF). These insignificant Q waves are produced as depolarization travels down the interventricular septum. The major flow of electricity is downward, but some electric impulses travel in a left-to-right direction. These smaller vectors point *away* from left sided surface electrodes. Therefore, the electrodes record a small negative deflection to their corresponding leads (the septal Q wave). Depolarization of the septum takes place within a span of 0.04 seconds. Prolongation of this value is one of the criteria that can be used to determine whether or not a Q wave is pathologic.

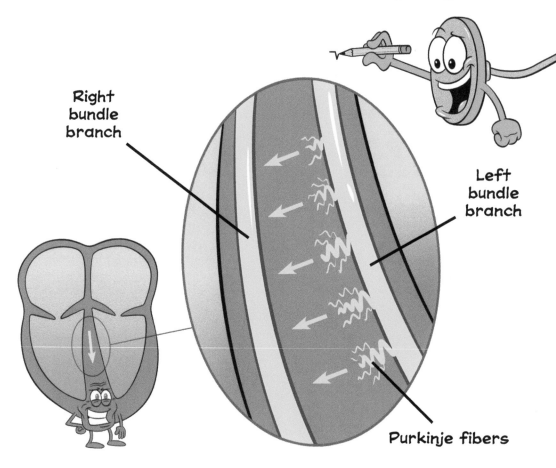

Right bundle branch

Left bundle branch

Purkinje fibers

We have discussed how MIs can be categorized with respect to the ST segment. The distinction of ST-elevation vs. non-ST-elevation MI is especially important in the acute setting when the ECG contains a wealth of clinically important information. MIs can also be categorized according to the presence or absence of pathologic Q waves, although this terminology is used less frequently.

Q Waves and Infarction

The distinction between Q wave MIs and non-Q wave MIs is of clinical relevance because pathologic Q waves are associated with a larger area of myocardial necrosis and a lower ejection fraction.

Cardiac magnetic resonance (CMR) and autopsy studies have demonstrated that transmural infarction (one involving the entire myocardium) and nontransmural infarction can both give rise to pathologic Q waves. Therefore, the presence of pathologic Q waves cannot be used to determine whether an infarct is transmural or nontransmural.

Septal Q waves are tiny because the electrode detects small vectors pointing toward it in the proximal myocardial wall. These vectors oppose the septal vectors pointing in the opposite direction. Pathologic Q waves develop because necrotic myocardial tissue is electrically neutral, lacking the vectors that usually face the electrode.

The infarct is an electric void that gives the electrode an unopposed view of the opposite wall. The vectors from the septum point away from the electrode, producing an abnormally large Q wave.

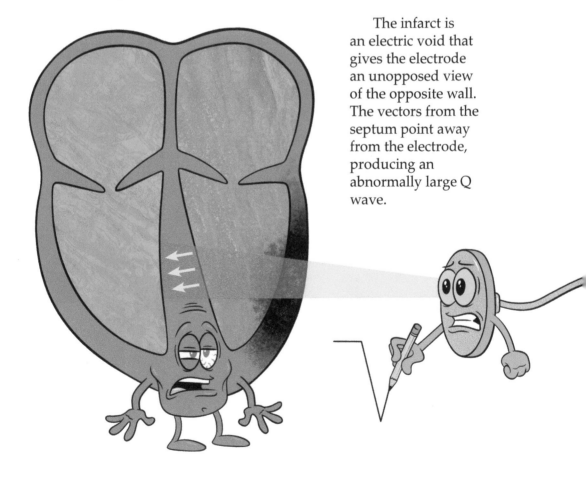

Poor R wave Progression

The R wave in the precordial leads normally undergoes a transition in morphology from short to tall when advancing from lead V1 to V6. Poor R wave progression (PRWP) refers to a change in this pattern, usually due to underlying cardiac pathology.

An abnormally low amplitude in leads V3 to V6 may suggest prior anteroseptal myocardial infarction. However, PRWP is a nonspecific finding that can also be caused by left ventricular hypertrophy, left bundle branch block, left anterior fascicular block, Wolff-Parkinson-White syndrome, dilated cardiomyopathy, dextrocardia, COPD, inaccurate chest electrode placement, or occur as a normal variant without association to cardiac or pulmonary disease.

Due to the multitude of possible etiologies for PRWP, it is not considered a useful finding for identifying patients with prior myocardial infarction. PRWP is often defined as an R wave amplitude < 3 mm in lead V3.

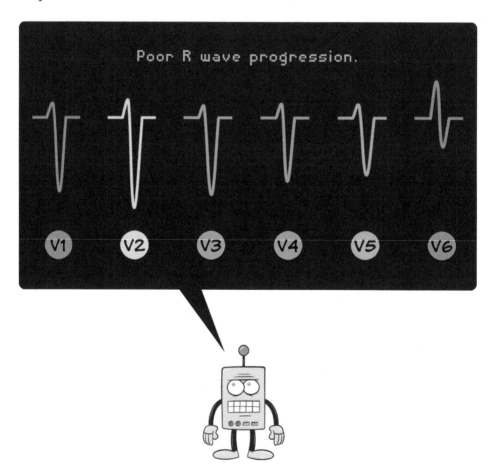

Let's quickly summarize the sequence of ECG changes following an acute MI. The first change to appear on the ECG is the development of hyperacute T waves. Several minutes later, ST segment elevation with reciprocal changes appear. Within hours, the T waves invert. Pathologic Q waves appear last and usually remain on the ECG as a permanent sign of infarction. As the process of infarction comes to an end, ST segment elevation returns to baseline and the T waves revert upright. The process of ECG normalization can take weeks to resolve. These changes, in combination with the patient's history, symptoms, and cardiac biomarkers, help estimate the age of an infarct.

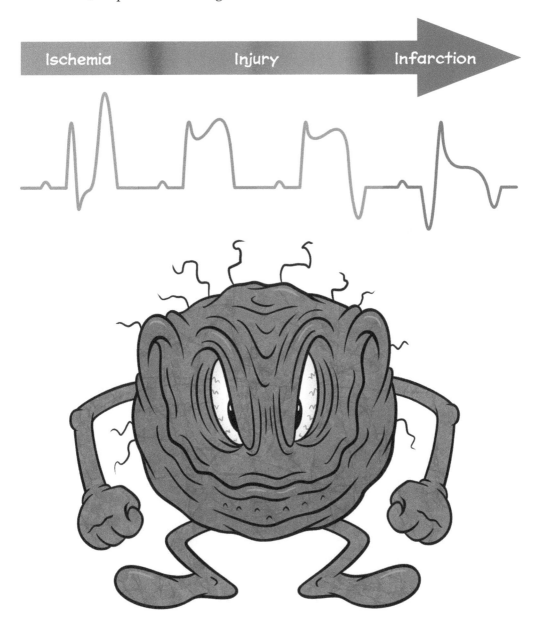

Localizing the Infarct

Once we have identified ST elevation or the presence of pathologic Q waves, an infarct can be localized to a specific region of the heart. Most infarcts involve the left ventricle. The ventricular myocardium is divided into regions called *walls* which correspond to the leads of the ECG. Anatomically adjacent leads are called *contiguous* leads. The characteristic ECG changes indicative of infarction appear in leads facing the infarct, while reciprocal changes occur in leads opposite the infarct.

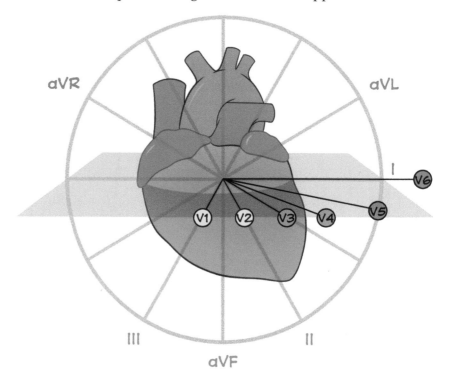

Walls/contiguous leads

I High Lateral	aVR	V1 Septal or posterior	V4 Anterior
II Inferior	aVL High Lateral	V2 Septal or posterior	V5 Lateral
III Inferior	aVF Inferior	V3 Anterior or posterior	V6 Lateral

Note: the posterior wall is indirectly visualized with reciprocal changes in the anteroseptal leads

It's common for an infarct to involve more than one anatomic lead grouping on the ECG because the coronary arteries usually supply multiple areas of the heart. Examples of infarct regions in combination include anteroseptal, anterolateral, and inferoposterior infarcts.

The location and amount of tissue that undergoes infarction depends on which coronary artery is occluded and the amount of collateral blood flow it provides. An understanding of coronary anatomy allows us to predict which coronary artery is blocked when reviewing an ECG with evidence of infarction.

- RCA = Right Coronary Artery
- PDA = Posterior Descending Artery
- LCx = Left Circumflex
- LAD = Left Anterior Descending

A more proximal arterial occlusion usually produces a larger area of infarction

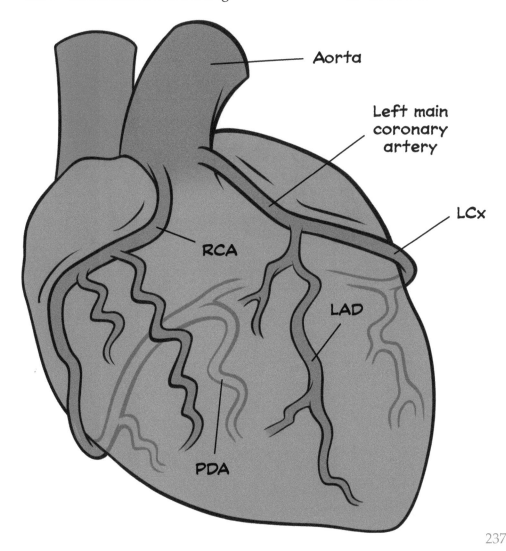

The left main coronary artery branches into the left anterior descending artery (LAD) and left circumflex artery (LCx). The LAD supplies the interventricular septum, anterior wall, and apex. The LCx wraps around the lateral aspect of the heart and supplies the lateral wall and high lateral wall superiorly.

The RCA gives off branches that supply the right ventricle. It also gives rise to the PDA. The PDA supplies the inferior and posterior walls. Although the PDA most commonly arises from the RCA, it sometimes arises from the LCx, or both.

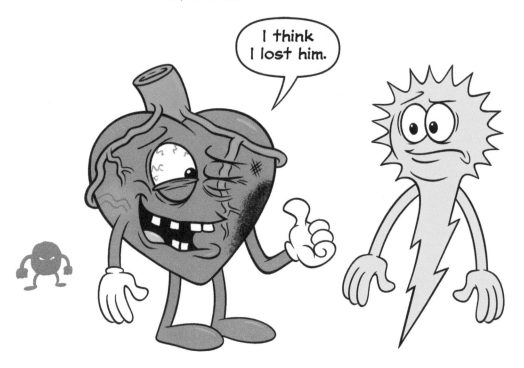

Likely culprit vessel **in relation to** location of infarct:

I	aVR	V1	V4
High lateral		Septal	Anterior
LCx		LAD	LAD
II	aVL	V2	V5
Inferior	High lateral	Septal	Lateral
RCA, LCx, PDA	LCx	LAD	LCx
III	aVF	V3	V6
Inferior	Inferior	Anterior	Lateral
RCA, LCx, PDA	RCA, LCx, PDA	LAD	LCx

Posterior / RCA, LCx, PDA: **reciprocal changes in V1 to V3**

Coronary Dominance

Variability in the origin of the PDA is expressed by the term *dominance*. Right dominant circulation is the most common type of coronary dominance, in which the right coronary artery gives rise to the PDA. Left dominant circulation occurs when the LCx gives rise to the PDA. A small percentage of people express a co-dominant circulation, in which the PDA is supplied by both the RCA and the LCx.

The chamber most vulnerable to a compromised blood supply is the left ventricle. It has the heaviest workload and its demand for oxygen is higher. Left coronary dominance therefore carries a greater risk of mortality compared with other types of dominance.

Right dominant circulation	Left dominant circulation	Co-dominant circulation
Very common	Less common	Relatively rare
PDA is supplied by RCA	PDA is supplied by LCx	PDA is supplied by RCA and LCx

The artery that supplies the PDA determines coronary dominance.

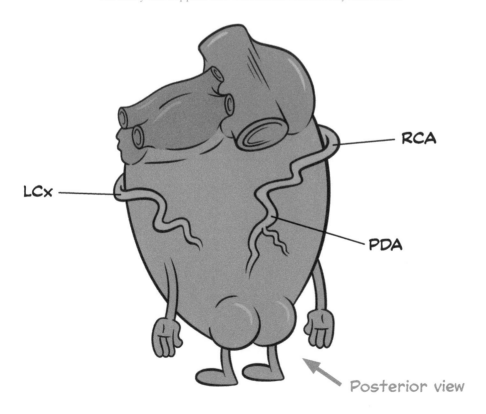

LCx

RCA

PDA

Posterior view

Anterior Wall Infarction

Anterior wall infarction is caused by an occlusion of the LAD. ECG changes indicative of infarction appear in leads V3 and V4. Unfortunately, an infarct in this region rarely presents in isolation. An anteroseptal MI involves the anterior wall and the septum, with ECG changes appearing in leads V1 to V4. An anterolateral MI involves the anterior wall and the lateral wall, with ECG changes in leads V3 to V6. An occlusion in the left main coronary artery results in an anteroseptal MI with lateral extension, which can include changes in V1 to V6, I and aVL. Lateral involvement may cause reciprocal changes in the inferior leads (II, III, and aVF). The LAD is also known as "the widow maker" because an anterior MI tends to involve a large area of the left ventricle and carries the worst prognosis of all the infarct locations.

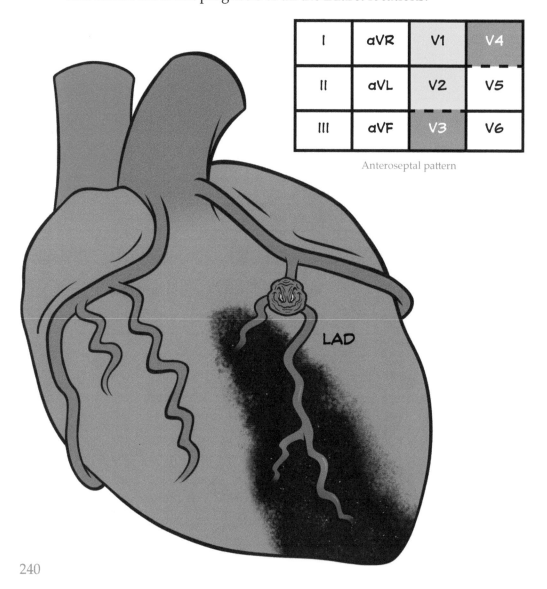

I	aVR	V1	V4
II	aVL	V2	V5
III	aVF	V3	V6

Anteroseptal pattern

LAD

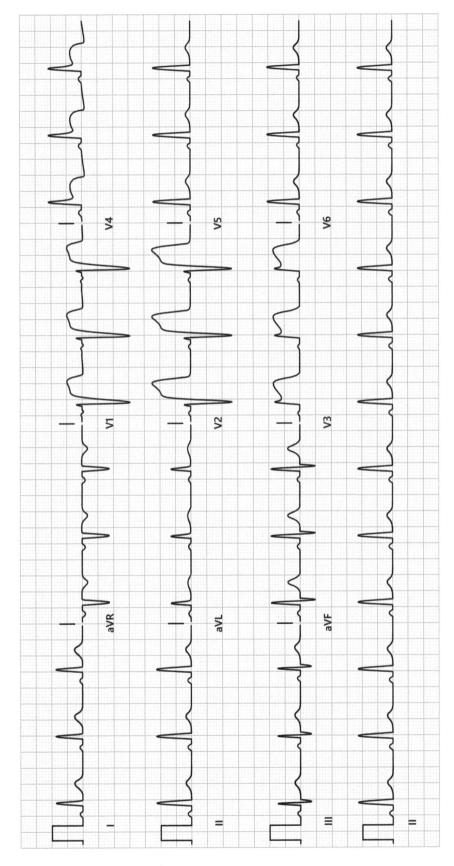

De Winter's Sign

De Winter's sign is considered an anterior STEMI equivalent and presents without obvious ST elevation. The pattern is indicative of an acute proximal LAD occlusion, occurring in approximately 2% of anterior STEMI cases. The de Winter ECG pattern is characterized by upsloping ST depression followed by tall, symmetrical, upright T waves in the precordial leads. Recognition of this pattern is clinically important because it presents without obvious ST elevation, which could lead to delayed or missed treatment.

Infarction in de Winter makes the T waves Spring and the ST segments Fall

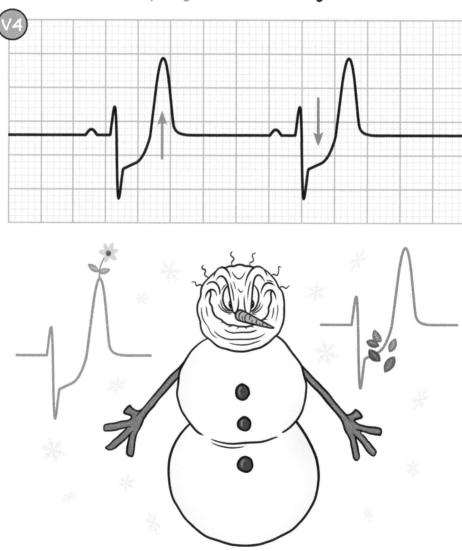

Wellens' Syndrome

Wellens' syndrome describes a collection of signs and symptoms suggesting critical stenosis of the LAD. Without urgent intervention, patients will develop an anterior wall MI within days to weeks. Wellens' syndrome is characterized by the appearance of biphasic or deeply inverted T waves in leads V2 and V3, recorded during a pain-free period in a patient with a history of angina.

The biphasic T wave pattern is known as type A, while the pattern of deep T wave inversion is known as type B. The type A pattern evolves into the type B pattern over time, and these T wave abnormalities are thought to occur due to unstable perfusion of the LAD.

Criteria:

- Intermittent chest pain
- Biphasic (type A) or deeply inverted (type B) T-waves in V2 and V3, possibly extending from V1 to V6
- Type A or type B pattern in a pain-free state
- Isoelectric or minimal ST deviation during chest pain
- Absence of pathologic Q waves in precordial leads
- Precordial R waves are preserved
- Normal or slightly elevated cardiac biomarkers

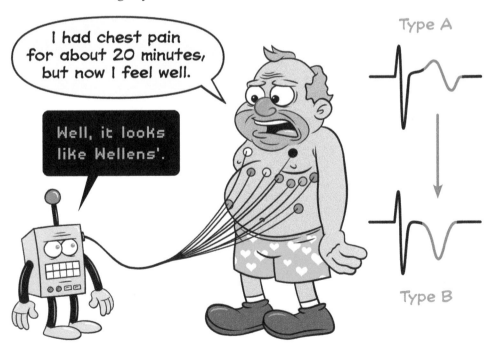

Lateral Wall Infarction

Infarction of the lateral wall is caused by an occlusion of the LCx. ECG changes appear in leads I and aVL (high lateral wall) and leads V5 and V6 (lateral wall proper). Reciprocal changes appear in the inferior leads (II, III, and aVF).

Lateral infarction can occur in combination with other infarct patterns, depending on the site of the coronary occlusion. As described in the previous section, an occlusion of the left main coronary artery can produce an anteroseptal MI with lateral extension.

If left coronary dominance is present, an occlusion of the LCx could produce an inferior-posterior-lateral wall MI.

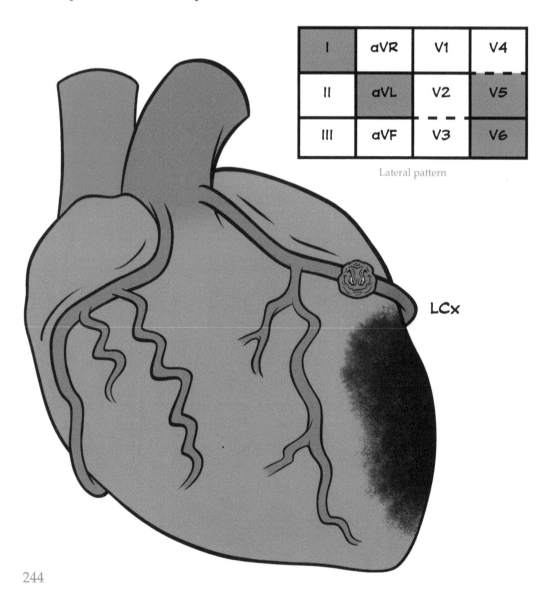

Lateral pattern

LCx

Lateral myocardial infarction

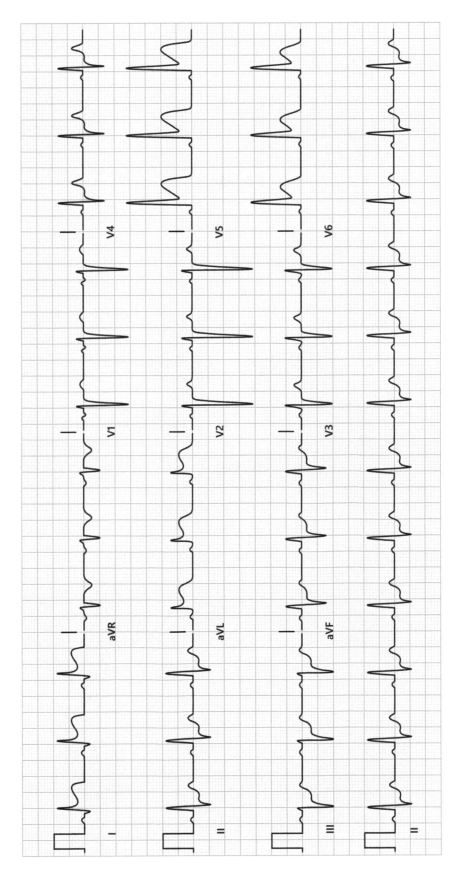

Inferior Wall Infarction

Myocardial infarction involving the inferior wall is commonly caused by an occlusion of the RCA or PDA in the setting of right coronary dominance.

ECG changes occur in leads II, III, and aVF. Reciprocal changes are seen in leads I and aVL, as well as in the anteroseptal leads. ST depression in leads V1 and V2 may indicate posterior wall involvement.

Inferolateral infarction is characterized by the presence of ST elevation in leads II, III, and aVF in combination with ST elevation in leads V5 and V6 or I and aVL. This pattern of infarction is indicative of left coronary dominance with the LCx as the likely culprit artery.

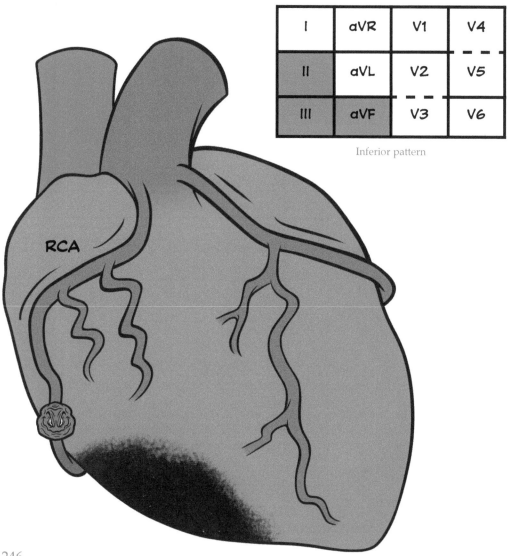

I	aVR	V1	V4
II	aVL	V2	V5
III	aVF	V3	V6

Inferior pattern

Inferior myocardial infarction

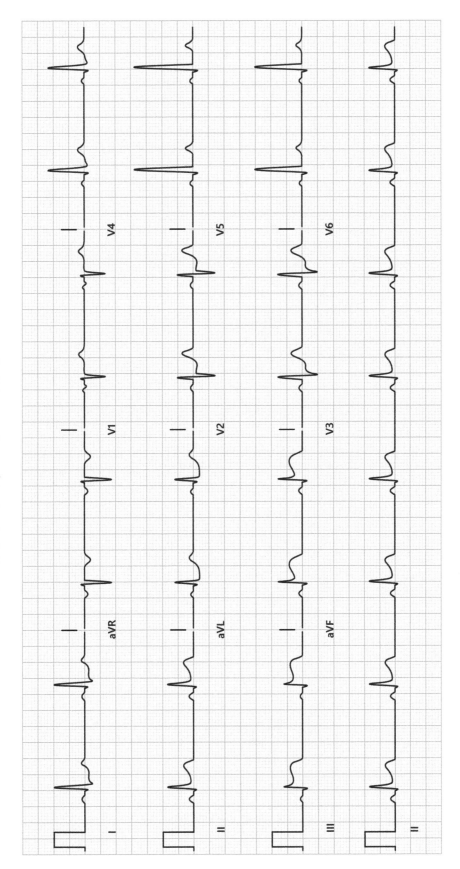

Posterior Wall Infarction

A posterior wall infarct occurs due to an occlusion of the RCA or PDA. It is often accompanied by infarction of the inferior wall due to their shared blood supply. Posterior wall infarction can also occur with lateral wall infarction in the context of left coronary dominance, in which the PDA is supplied by the LCx.

The conventional 12 lead ECG lead does not provide a direct view of the posterior wall. The presence of ST depression in leads V1 to V3 suggests infarction and represents reciprocal changes from the posterior wall. Tall, broad R waves may also be seen in V1 to V3, analogous to the pathologic Q waves of infarction.

The placement of electrodes to create posterior leads (V7 to V9) may help with the diagnosis of a posterior infarct. ST elevation of 0.5 mm or more in these leads indicates posterior wall infarction.

The posterior leads are positioned on the same horizontal plane as V6. Lead V7 is placed at the left posterior axillary line, V8 at the tip of the scapula, and V9 at the left paraspinal border.

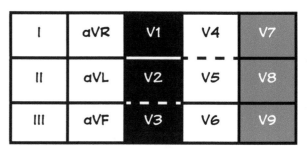

I	aVR	V1	V4	V7
II	aVL	V2	V5	V8
III	aVF	V3	V6	V9

Posterior pattern

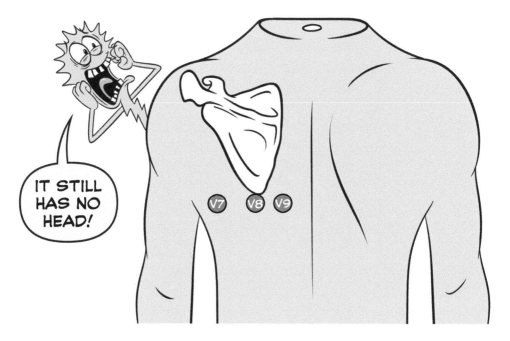

IT STILL HAS NO HEAD!

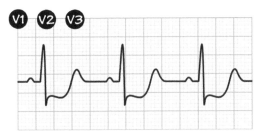

Tall R waves and ST segment depression

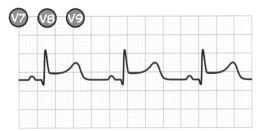

ST segment elevation ≥ 0.5 mm

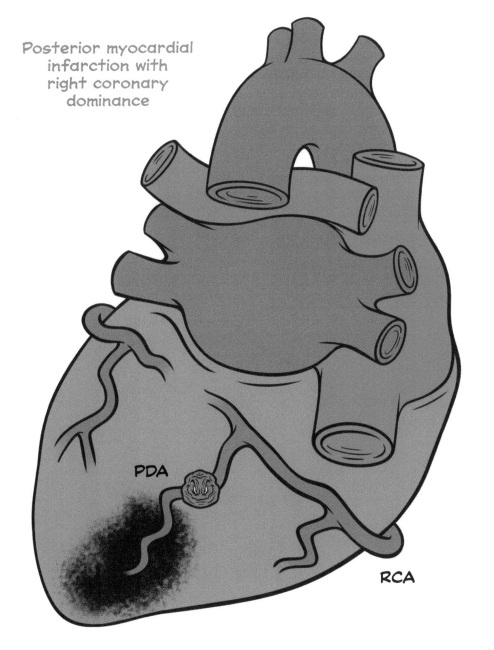

Posterior myocardial infarction with right coronary dominance

PDA

RCA

Right Ventricular (RV) Infarction

Right ventricular infarction is caused by an occlusion of the proximal RCA and complicates up to 50% of inferior myocardial infarctions. The area of infarction can also extend to the posterior wall. Systemic hypotension may develop if the deteriorating right ventricle is unable to sufficiently pump blood through the pulmonary circuit to the left ventricle. Nitrates are contraindicated due to the risk severe hypotension, which is treated with fluid loading.

RV infarction is suggested by ST elevation in lead V1 and ST elevation in lead III greater than in lead II. A RV infarct can be confirmed by using right-sided leads. Electrodes are placed on the right side of the chest in a mirror image configuration relative to the standard left-sided electrode placement. These leads are named V1R through V6R. Lead V4R is the most sensitive and specific for diagnosing RV infarction, and sometimes it may be the only right-sided lead obtained. It is placed in the right 5th intercostal space in the midclavicular line.

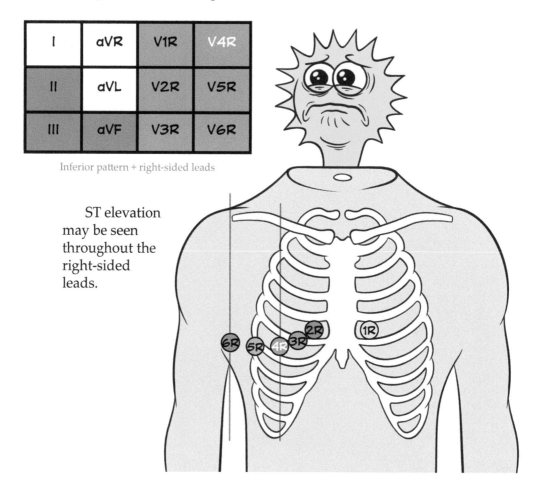

Inferior pattern + right-sided leads

ST elevation may be seen throughout the right-sided leads.

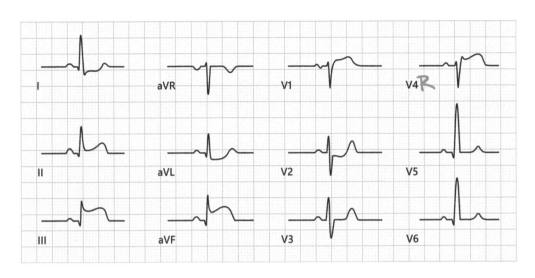

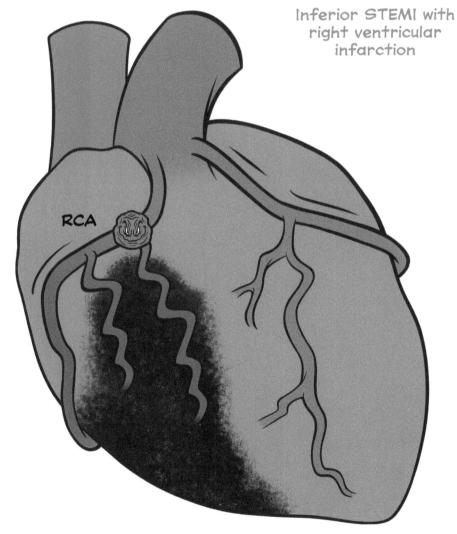

Inferior STEMI with
right ventricular
infarction

RCA

STEMI in the Presence of LBBB or Paced Rhythm

A LBBB or paced rhythm makes the diagnosis of infarction on the ECG difficult. These conditions cause ST segment deviation that mimic or mask acute infarction. However, a set of guidelines known as the *Smith-modified Sgarbossa criteria* were developed to accurately diagnose an acute coronary occlusion in the presence of LBBB.

These criteria rely on the concept of *concordance* and *discordance*, which describe the relationship of the ST segment relative to the predominant deflection of the QRS complex. Concordance refers to ST segment deviation in the same direction as the predominant QRS deflection. Discordance refers to ST segment deviation that moves in the direction opposite to the predominant QRS deflection.

Smith-modified Sgarbossa criteria

- Concordant ST elevation ≥ 1 mm in any lead
- Concordant ST depression ≥ 1 mm in leads V1, V2, or V3
- Discordance in any lead in which the amplitude of ST elevation is greater than 1/4 of the S wave amplitude

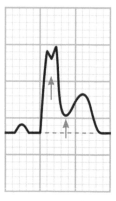
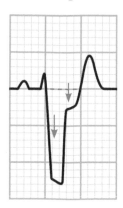
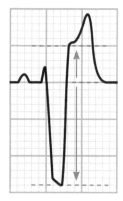

Positive concordance ≥ 1mm (any lead)　Negative concordance ≥ 1mm (V1-V3)　Excessive discordance (any lead)

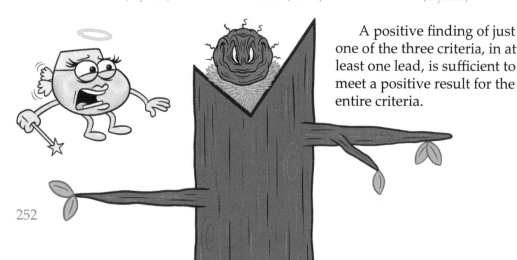

A positive finding of just one of the three criteria, in at least one lead, is sufficient to meet a positive result for the entire criteria.

Arrhythmias and Myocardial Infarction

Myocardial infarction causes severe metabolic and electrophysiological imbalances that can lead to the development of a wide range of conduction disturbances, including malignant ventricular arrhythmias.

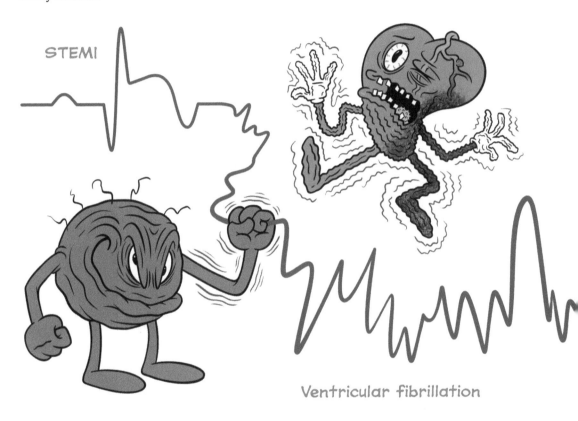

STEMI

Ventricular fibrillation

In the post-infarction period, persistent sinus tachycardia increases myocardial oxygen demand and carries an increased mortality risk. Atrial fibrillation also carries a poor prognosis as it is associated with extensive myocardial damage, heart failure, and stroke.

Bradyarrhythmias commonly appear with inferior wall infarction due to increased activity of the parasympathetic nervous system. If severe, sinus bradycardia can lead to hypotension and shock. First-degree AV block and Mobitz type I (Wenckebach) AV block are also commonly seen with inferior wall infarction and are usually transient.

Mobitz type II AV block is most commonly associated with anterior wall infarction and carries a high risk of progressing to complete heart block. Anterior wall infarction also strongly correlates with RBBB, LBBB, bifascicular block, and trifascicular block.

Reperfusion Therapy

Left heart catheterization allows for the visualization of the coronary arteries. Reperfusion therapy restores blood flow as soon as possible to prevent the ischemic myocardium from dying. Percutaneous coronary intervention (PCI) or fibrinolysis may be used to treat an occluded coronary artery. PCI is preferred to fibrinolysis, which is usually recommended when PCI cannot be performed in a timely manner.

PCI is ideally performed in 90 minutes or less from the point of medical contact, known as the "door-to-balloon time." If a patient arrives at a non-PCI capable hospital, then the door-to-balloon time should be 120 minutes or less with transfer to a PCI-capable hospital.

Primary PCI consists of using coronary catheterization to perform a balloon angioplasty. During this procedure a thin metal guidewire is introduced into the coronary artery, past the atherosclerotic plaque and occlusive thrombus. A catheter equipped with a deflated balloon is advanced over the guidewire and positioned at the site of the occlusion. The balloon is then inflated to compress the plaque and open the obstruction. The balloon is then deflated and removed with the catheter and guidewire.

In some cases a metal stent attached to the deflated balloon catheter is introduced into the culprit artery. After the balloon is positioned at the site of occlusion and inflated, the stent expands to remain permanently in place. Coronary blood flow is restored, thereby relieving the ischemia.

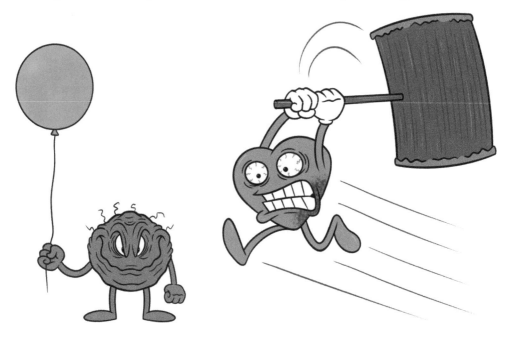

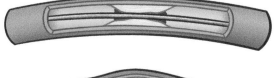

A guidewire is advanced through the stenotic plaque and thrombus.

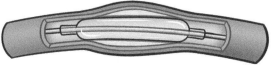

A balloon catheter is introduced and inflated, which compresses and opens the obstruction.

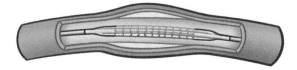

A balloon catheter carrying a stent is positioned in the opening.

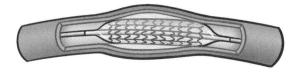

The stent is deployed with inflation of the balloon.

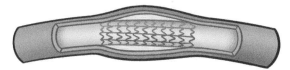

The catheter and guidewire are removed and the stent remains permanently in place.

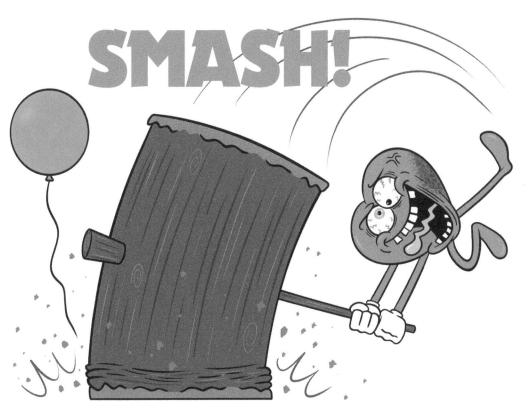

Pericarditis

Acute pericarditis is an inflammation of the sac-like membrane surrounding the heart. The condition most commonly has a viral etiology, but may also be caused by bacteria, malignancy, or other sources of inflammation. Pericarditis is characterized by sharp, pleuritic chest pain that improves when sitting up and leaning forward, and worsens when lying supine. Auscultation of a pericardial friction rub is highly specific for acute pericarditis, but is not always present on physical examination.

Acute pericarditis causes widespread ST elevation and PR depression with reciprocal changes in leads V1 and aVR. Unlike myocardial infarction, it does not produce pathologic Q waves. There are four classic stages that describe the sequence of ECG changes in pericarditis:

1. Diffuse ST elevation and PR depression with reciprocal changes in leads aVR and V1.
2. Normalization of ST segment and progressive T wave flattening.
3. T wave inversion.
4. Complete normalization.

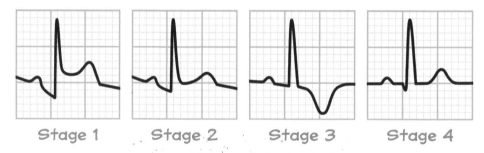

Stage 1   Stage 2   Stage 3   Stage 4

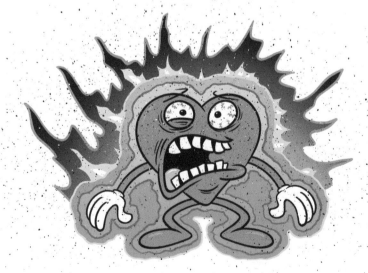

Spodik's sign is an ECG change that favors the diagnosis pericarditis. It is characterized by a down-sloping *TP segment* during stage 1. Spodik's sign is best visualized in leads II, V5, and V6.

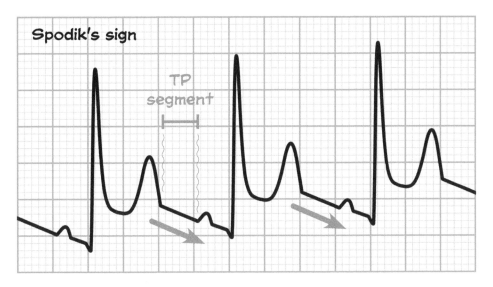

Another way to distinguish acute pericarditis from acute myocardial infarction is to analyze the morphology of the ST elevation. Pericarditis tends to produce a smiley shape (concave), while infarction is more likely to produce a frowny shape (convex).

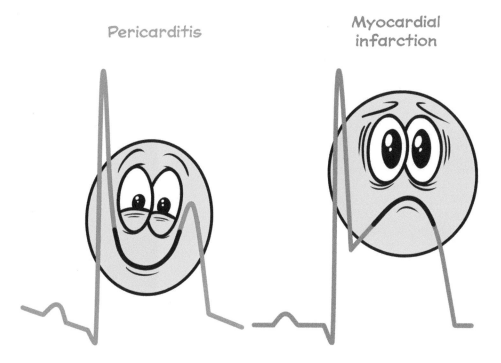

Brugada Syndrome

Brugada syndrome is an inherited disorder that can cause sudden cardiac death in people with structurally normal hearts. The underlying pathophysiology of Brugada syndrome involves a genetic defect that results in dysfunctional sodium ion channels. Thus, the disorder is referred to as a type of *channelopathy*.

Sudden cardiac death may occur due to the development of malignant ventricular arrhythmias, such as polymorphic VT or ventricular fibrillation. These episodes typically occur during sleep or at rest. Brugada syndrome is most commonly seen in adult men of Asian descent, and the condition is inherited as an autosomal dominant trait.

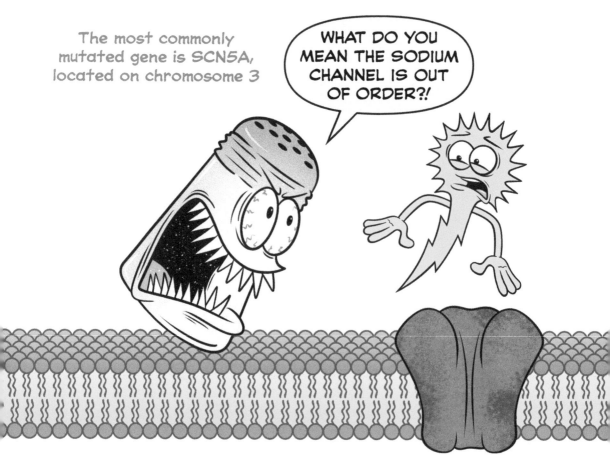

Brugada syndrome consists of ECG changes involving elevation of the ST segment in conjunction with symptoms related to life-threatening arrhythmias. Patients that are found to have the typical ECG findings without symptoms are said to have the *Brugada pattern*, rather than Brugada syndrome.

The distinct patterns of ST elevation seen in Brugada syndrome may be intermittent or concealed. The infusion of a sodium channel blocker, such as flecainide or procainamide, can unmask a concealed ECG pattern and aid in the diagnosis of Brugada syndrome. There are two distinct patterns of ST elevation. The diagnosis of Brugada syndrome requires a type 1 or type 2 pattern in lead V1 or V2 **in combination** with at least one of the Brugada criteria.

Brugada criteria:

- Documented case of polymorphic VT
- History of syncope
- Family history of sudden death at less than 45 years of age
- Brugada type 1 pattern in a family member
- Induced VT during electrophysiology study
- Nocturnal agonal respiration

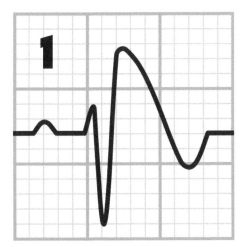 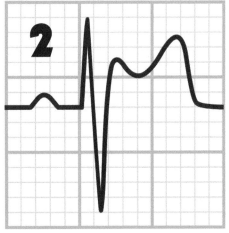

The **type 1 pattern** lacks a distinct R' wave. There is coved ST elevation of at least 2 mm in lead V1 or V2. The ST segment drops down like a ski slope into a symmetrically negative T wave.

The **type 2 pattern** has an RSr' configuration, with a "saddleback" morphology in lead V1 or V2. The r' is at least 2mm tall.

Recognizing Brugada syndrome can be life-saving. The definitive treatment of Brugada syndrome is ICD placement.

Takotsubo Cardiomyopathy

Takotsubo cardiomyopathy, also known as broken heart syndrome, apical ballooning syndrome, and stress-induced cardiomyopathy, is a syndrome that mimics myocardial infarction. The presentation includes chest pain, ST segment elevation and depression, T wave inversion, and even elevated cardiac biomarkers. However, patients are found to have normal coronary arteries if they are taken to the cath lab for intervention.

Takotsubo is characterized by weakening and ballooning of the left ventricle, usually as a result of severe physical or emotional stress, such as the loss of a loved one (hence the name broken heart syndrome). The word "takotsubo" is a Japanese term for a pot used to catch octopuses, which the left ventricle resembles as it contracts and balloons out.

Elderly females are most commonly affected by the condition which tends to resolve in a few weeks. The pathogenesis of takotsubo cardiomyopathy is not well understood, but catecholamine excess during times of stress is postulated to play a role.

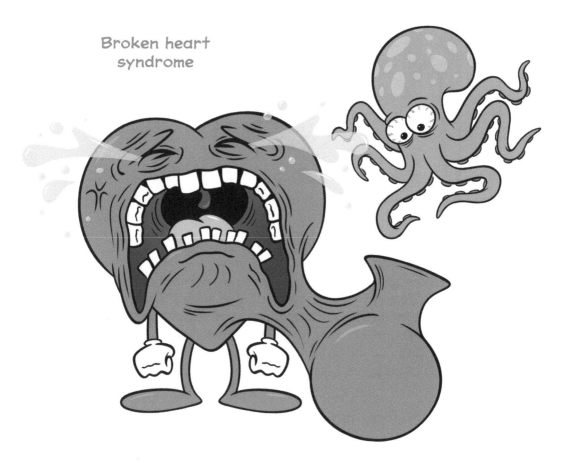

Broken heart
syndrome

Prinzmetal Angina

Prinzmetal angina, also known as vasospastic angina, is characterized by episodes of chest pain at rest caused by coronary artery spasm. The condition causes a pattern of ECG changes that resembles a STEMI, including ST elevation with reciprocal ST depression.

Unlike a STEMI, the ECG changes are transient and typically normalize with the resolution of chest pain. The ST elevation is reversible with the use of vasodilators such as nitroglycerin or calcium channel blockers.

Coronary artery spasm

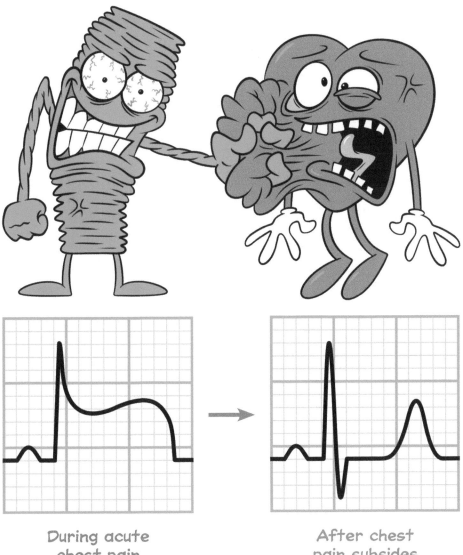

During acute
chest pain

After chest
pain subsides

Early Repolarization

Early repolarization is an ECG pattern of widespread ST segment elevation. It is generally considered benign and usually found as an incidental finding in young, healthy males. However, some studies have linked the pattern to a risk of sudden cardiac death. Early repolarization presents a diagnostic challenge because it may mimic an acute MI or pericarditis. These conditions can be distinguished from each other with the recognition of some characteristic ECG findings.

In early repolarization there is either slurring or notching at the terminal end of the QRS complex in two or more contiguous leads. The notched morphology is also known as the "fish hook" pattern, often seen in lead V4. Reciprocal changes typical of an acute MI are absent in early repolarization. Furthermore, the ST elevation that's seen with early repolarization remains fairly stable over time. This is in contrast to infarction, in which ST deviations evolve rather quickly.

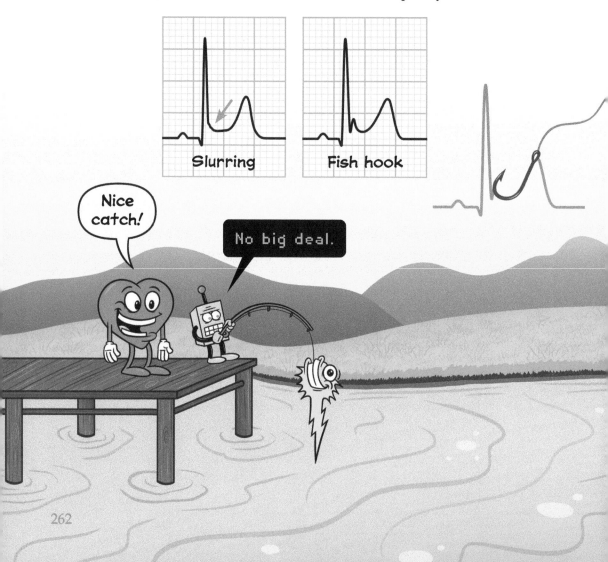

Sparkson's Summary: Chapter 9

- Occlusion of a coronary artery causes myocardial ischemia, injury, and infarction.

- ECG changes following an acute MI: hyperacute T waves, ST elevation, reciprocal ST depression, T wave inversions, and pathologic Q waves.

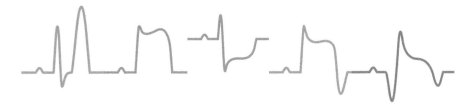

- Anterior wall infarction: occlusion of the LAD results in ECG changes in leads V3 and V4, and leads V1 and V2 if there involvement of the septum.

- Lateral wall infarction: occlusion of the LCx results in ECG changes in the leads I, aVL, V5, and V6. Reciprocal changes appear in the inferior leads (II, III, and aVF).

- Inferior wall infarction: occlusion of the RCA or PDA results in ECG changes in leads II, III, and aVF. Reciprocal changes appear in leads I and aVL, as well as in the anteroseptal leads.

- Posterior wall infarction: occlusion of the RCA or PDA results in ECG changes in leads V1 to V3 and V7 to V9 (posterior leads).

- Right ventricular infarction: occlusion of the proximal RCA results in ST elevation in lead V1, ST elevation in lead III greater than in lead II, and ST elevation in lead V4R (right-sided chest lead).

I High Lateral	aVR	V1 Septal or posterior	V4 Anterior
II Inferior	aVL High Lateral	V2 Septal or posterior	V5 Lateral
III Inferior	aVF Inferior	V3 Anterior or posterior	V6 Lateral

- Acute coronary syndrome includes: unstable angina, NSTEMI, and STEMI.

- Poor R wave progression may result from underlying cardiac patholgy, but the finding is nonspecific.

- De Winter's sign: STEMI equivalent consisting of upsloping ST depression followed by tall, symmetrical, upright T waves in the precordial leads.

- Wellens' syndrome: suggests critical stenosis of the LAD consisting of biphasic or deeply inverted T waves in leads V2 and V3, recorded during a pain-free period in a patient with a history of angina.

- Myocardial infarction can lead to life-threatening arrhythmias.

- The "door-to-balloon time" for PCI is 90 minutes or less from the point of medical contact at a PCI-capable hospital, or 120 minutes or less if the patient needs to be transferred to a PCI-capable hospital.

- Pericarditis: inflammation of the pericardium results in diffuse ST elevation and PR depression with reciprocal changes in leads aVR and V1.

- Brugada syndrome: an inherited channelopathy with distinct ECG patterns in leads V1 or V2, in combination with a sign or symptom listed in the Brugada criteria. Brugada syndrome carries a risk of sudden cardiac death and is treated with ICD implantation.

- Takotsubo cardiomyopathy: weakening and ballooning of the left ventricle causes chest pain, ECG changes, and elevated cardiac biomarkers. It is referred to as a stress-induced cardiomyopathy with normal coronaries upon evaluation in the cath lab.

- Prinzmetal angina: chest pain caused coronary artery spasm with transient ECG changes resembling a STEMI.

- Early repolarization: diffuse ST elevation with slurring or notching at the terminal end of the QRS complex; generally considered benign.

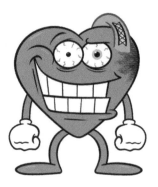
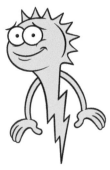

CHAPTER 10

THE WILDCARD CHAPTER

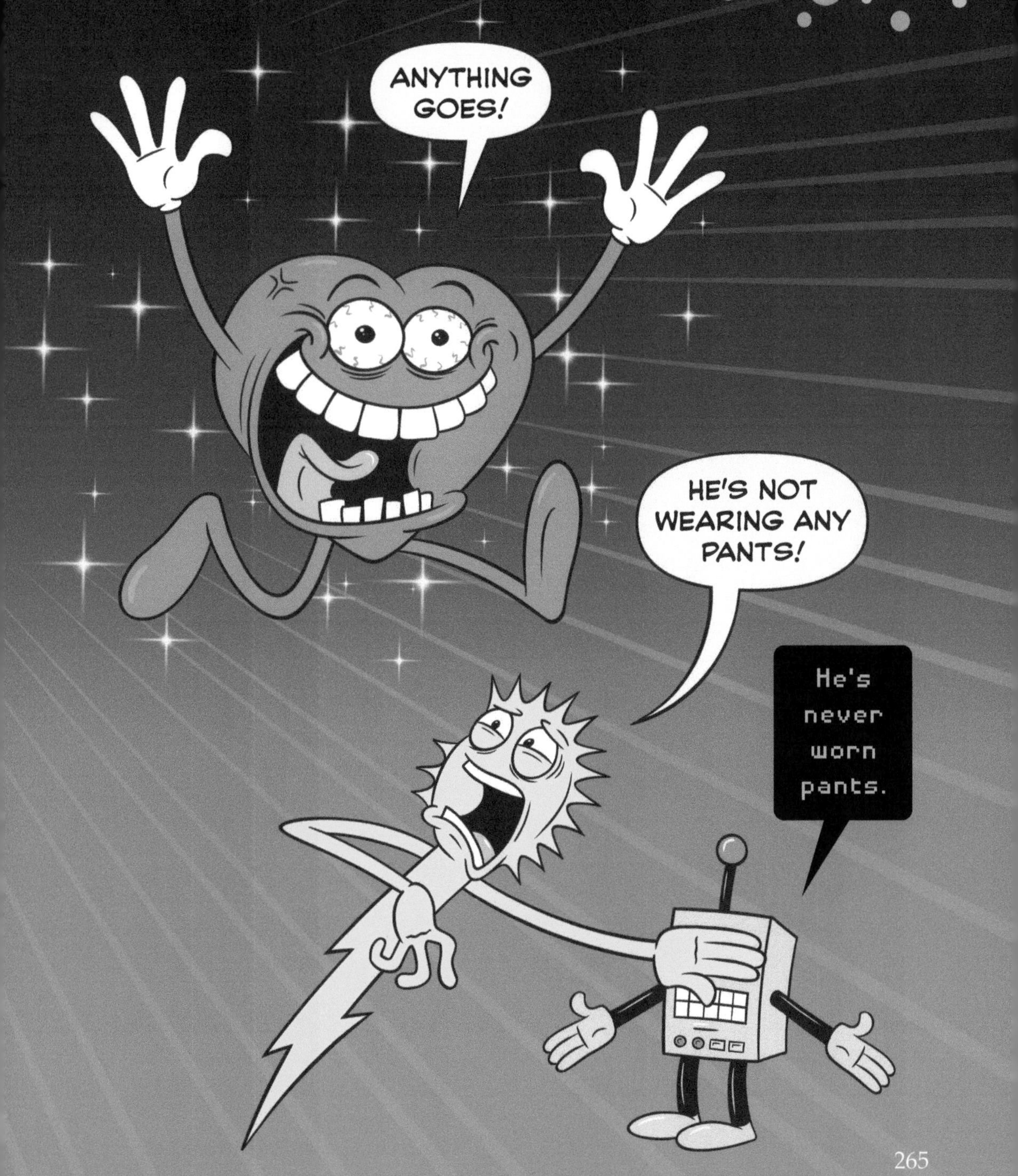

Hyperkalemia

The normal serum potassium (K⁺) level is between 3.5 to 5.0 mEq/L. Severe elevation of the serum potassium level causes a sequence of ECG changes that may culminate with ventricular fibrillation and death. Marked elevation of serum potassium warrants a repeat blood test to confirm the finding and rule out pseudohyperkalemia. Manifestations of hyperkalemia on the ECG include the appearance of peaked T waves, prolongation of the PR interval, QRS complex widening, and the flattening and disappearance of P waves.

Serum potassium mEq/L	5.5 to 6.5	6.5 to 8	8 to 10	> 10
Common ECG findings	Tall, peaked T waves	QRS complex widening and PR interval lengthening	P waves flatten and disappear	QRS complex merges with T wave to form sine wave

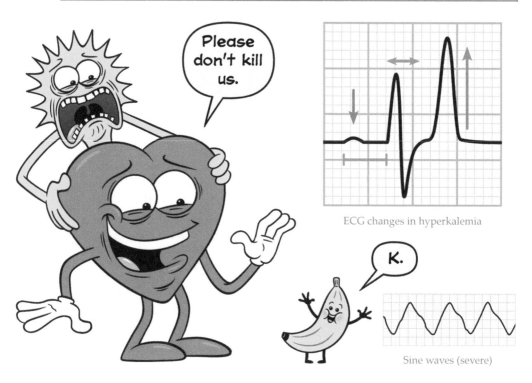

ECG changes in hyperkalemia

Sine waves (severe)

Hypokalemia

Hypokalemia is defined as a serum potassium ion level less than 3.5 mEq/L. Significant hypokalemia may cause supraventricular tachyarrhythmias and has the potential to provoke malignant ventricular arrhythmias. ECG changes most commonly appear when the serum K^+ level drops below 2.7 mEq/L.

The ECG changes of hypokalemia include ST segment depression, T wave flattening and inversion, and the development of prominent U waves. Severe hypokalemia causes the T and U waves to fuse, creating an *apparent* long QT interval (referred to as a long QU interval). Prolongation of the PR interval may also be seen.

This ECG pattern increases the risk of a premature beat causing the R on T phenomenon. Hypokalemia is often seen in conjunction with hypomagnesemia (low magnesium), which is also associated with a prolonged QT interval and the development of torsades de pointes.

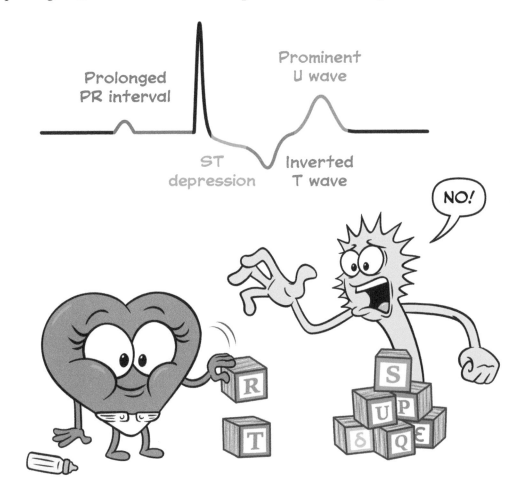

Calcium Disorders

The normal serum calcium (Ca^{2+}) level is between 8.5 to 10.5 mg/dL (2.2 to 2.6 mmol/L). *Hypercalcemia* accelerates ventricular repolarization, which shortens the QT interval. The most common causes of hypercalcemia are hyperparathyroidism and malignancy. In contrast, *hypocalcemia* prolongs the QT interval. As with hypokalemia and hypomagnesemia, prolongation of the QT interval in hypocalcemia increases the risk of torsades de pointes. The most common causes of hypocalcemia are hypoparathyroidism, vitamin D deficiency, and renal disease.

Hypercalcemia: Ca^{2+} greater than 10.5 mg/dL

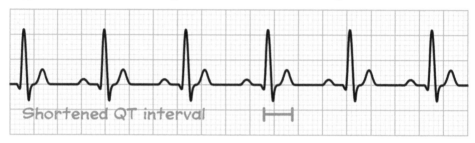

Hypocalcemia: Ca^{2+} less than 8.5 mg/dL

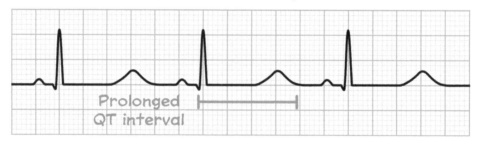

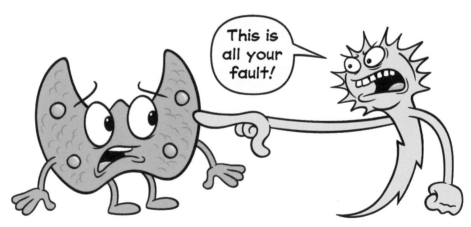

DRUGS

The Effect of Drugs on Conduction

A variety of cardiac and non-cardiac drugs can influence the electrical conduction system. The mechanism is through either a direct effect on myocardial ion channels or by altering autonomic nervous system input to the heart. The figure below illustrates the relationship between a normal ventricular action potential and an ECG tracing.

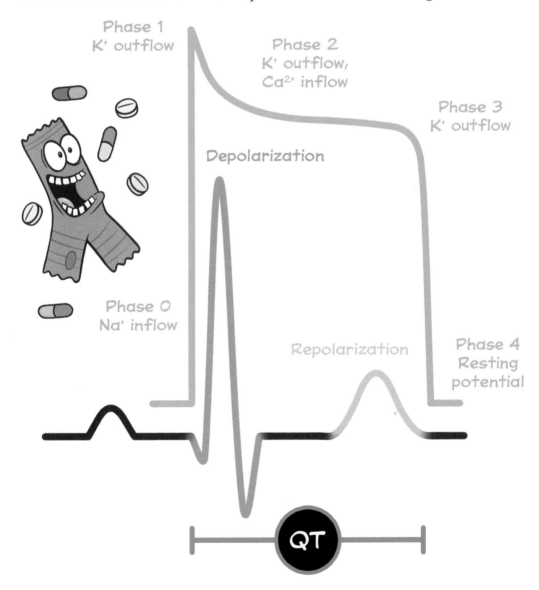

The QT interval corresponds to the duration of the ventricular action potential. As you can see from the schematic above, the QT interval is vulnerable to prolongation if certain drugs interfere with the delicate balance of inward and outward ion currents.

269

Drugs with antiarrhythmic properties are grouped according to the *Vaughan-Williams classification system*. There are four major classes based on the drug's predominant ion channel and receptor effects. However, most antiarrhythmic drugs have more than one action.

Class I drugs are the sodium channel blockers, which are subdivided into classes IA, IB, and IC. Class II consists of the beta blockers, class III contains the potassium channel blockers, and class IV drugs contains the calcium channel blockers.

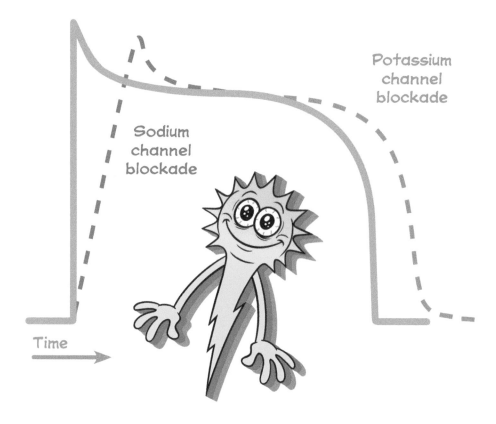

Let's review a couple of mechanisms by which antiarrhythmic drugs can terminate a reentrant arrhythmia. Sodium channel blockade reduces the rate at which phase 0 of the action potential rises, slowing conduction. Slowing the speed of a retrograde impulse can block it from engaging in a reentry circuit.

Potassium channel blockers lengthen the duration of phase 3 of the action potential, and thus prolong the refractory period. By extending the refractory period, a retrograde impulse may reach nonexcitable tissue and get extinguished before entering a reentry circuit. Unfortunately, in some conditions these same mechanisms can promote dangerous arrhythmias, rather than terminate them.

Class I (Sodium Channel Blockers)

Class IA drugs have a moderate inhibitory effect on phase 0 of the action potential. In addition, they have a mild class III drug effect and prolong repolarization during phase 3. These agents prolong the QT interval which may increase the risk of developing polymorphic VT. Quinidine is used infrequently due to its negative side effect profile.

Class IB drugs such as lidocaine, phenytoin, and mexiletine express their electrophysiologic effects only at rapid heart rates (e.g. during a tachyarrhythmia). Inhibition of the fast sodium current is weak and the duration of the action potential is shortened. Therefore, QT prolongation does not occur. Class IB agents act selectively on diseased tissue to facilitate the interruption of reentry circuits.

Class IC drugs are the strongest Na⁺ channel blockers, which significantly slow electrical conduction and cause QRS complex widening. They are frequently used to control supraventricular tachyarrhythmias such as atrial fibrillation. Na⁺ channel blockers have also been known to unmask the Brugada ECG pattern in susceptible individuals, although the clinical significance of this in asymptomatic patients is not well established.

Class	Na⁺ channel effect	Repolarization time	Drugs
IA	Moderate inhibition	Prolongs	Quinidine, disopyramide, procainamide
IB	Weak inhibition	Shortens	Lidocaine, phenytoin, mexiletine
IC	Major inhibition	No effect	Flecainide, propafenone

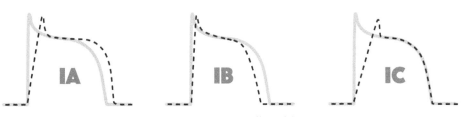

Dotted lines represent effect of drug

Class II (Beta Blockers)

Beta blockers inhibit beta adrenergic receptors and suppress sympathetic nervous system activity. This causes a decrease in heart rate and prolongation of the PR interval.

Beta blockers depress the slope of phase 4 of the pacemaker action potential, thereby increasing the time required to reach the depolarization threshold. The pacemaker current during phase 4 is called the *funny current* and is designated I_f. Beta blockers inhibit I_f, which results in decreased SA node automaticity and prolonged AV node conduction.

Class II antiarrhythmics are frequently used to treat supraventricular and ventricular tachyarrhythmias. Propranolol, acebutolol, and sotalol are examples of beta blockers approved by the U.S. Food and Drug Administration for antiarrhythmic use. Sotalol also has class III effects.

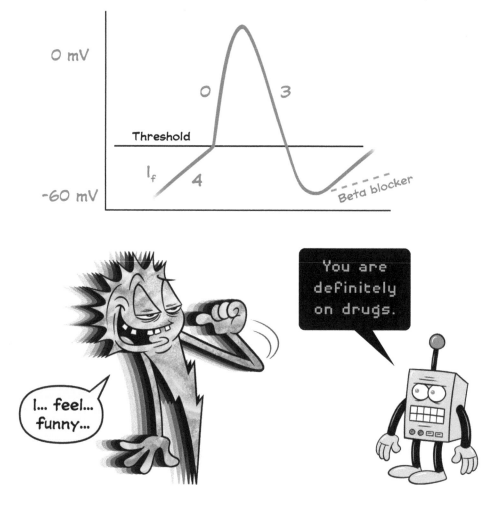

Class III (Potassium Channel Blockers)

Class III drugs block outward potassium currents, prolonging phase 3 of the action potential and the effective refractory period. Potassium channel blockers prolong the PR, QRS, and QT intervals. They are commonly used to treat supraventricular and ventricular arrhythmias.

Examples of class III agents include ibutilide, dofetilide, sotalol, and amiodarone. Sotalol is a mixed class II and class III agent. Amiodarone is mainly a class III drug, but also has class I, II, and IV effects.

All class III drugs have proarrhythmic potential. *Proarrhythmia* refers to the provocation of an arrhythmia, paradoxically, by antiarrhythmic drug therapy.

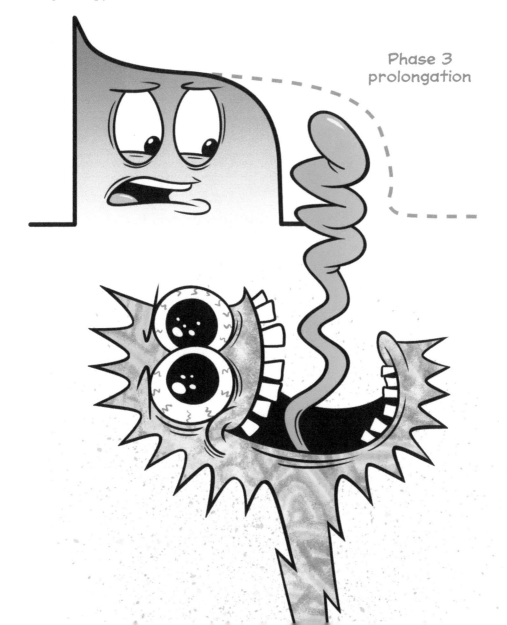

Phase 3 prolongation

Class IV (Calcium Channel Blockers) and Adenosine

Verapamil and diltiazem are class IV drugs known as non-dihydropyridine calcium channel blockers. These agents prolong both the cardiac conduction time and the refractory period in the AV node. They are used in the treatment of atrial fibrillation and can terminate or prevent paroxysmal supraventricular tachycardia.

Amlodipine and nifedipine are known as dihydropyridine calcium channel blockers. They do not have significant electrophysiologic effects and are primarily used in the treatment of hypertension.

Adenosine is an uncategorized antiarrhythmic drug used as a first-line agent to terminate reentrant arrhythmias involving the AV node.

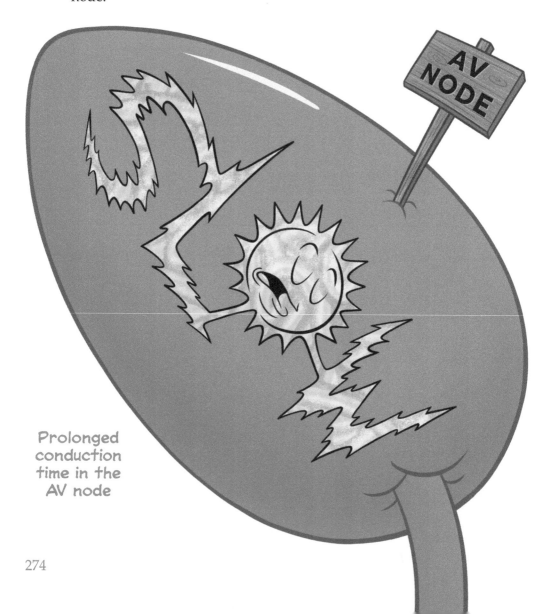

Prolonged conduction time in the AV node

Digoxin

Digoxin is used in the treatment of systolic heart failure and atrial fibrillation. The drug provides an increase in vagal tone without decreasing contractility, as can occur with beta blockers or calcium channel blockers.

Therapeutic doses of digoxin produces characteristic changes on the ECG, known as the "digoxin effect." The characteristic features include down-sloping ST segment depression with a scooped appearance. There may also be T wave flattening or inversion and shortening of the QT interval. The digoxin effect does not indicate digoxin toxicity; it's simply a sign that the drug is being taken.

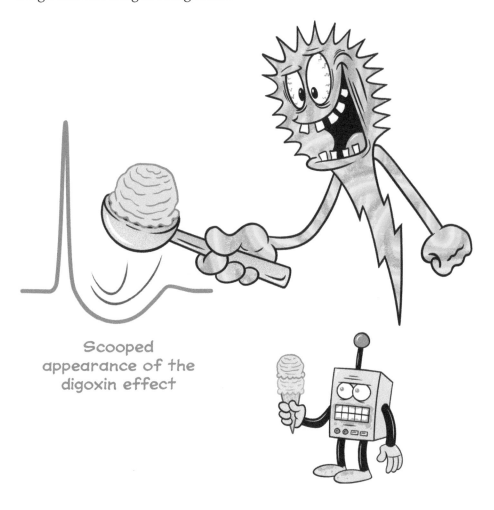

Scooped
appearance of the
digoxin effect

Digoxin has a very narrow therapeutic range and toxicity can provoke almost any type of arrhythmia. The classic arrhythmia associated with digoxin toxicity is PAT with block.

Nitrates

Nitrates are vasodilators that are commonly prescribed to treat angina, or chest pain, related to blocked or constricted vessels in the heart. Nitrates produce antianginal and anti-ischemic effects by decreasing myocardial oxygen demand through coronary and systemic vasodilation. The relaxation and dilation of blood vessels increases the delivery of oxygen-rich blood to the heart and reduces stress to the left ventricular wall during systole.

Headache due to meningeal arterial dilation is the most common side effect of nitrates. Nitrate-induced hypotension is also common, but patients are often asymptomatic.

Nitrates reduce preload to the heart and are contraindicated in the setting of right ventricular infarction. Patients with right ventricular infarction can develop severe hypotension in response to nitrates due to poor contractility of the right ventricle. The administration of nitrates is also contraindicated with concurrent use of phosphodiesterase-5 inhibitors for the treatment of erectile dysfunction. This combination of medications can lead to profound hypotension or even death.

Common nitrate preparations include sublingual nitroglycerin, nitroglycerin spray, transdermal nitroglycerin, isosorbide mononitrate, and isosorbide dinitrate. Sublingual nitroglycerin is the treatment of choice for acute angina or for prophylaxis prior to activities known to exacerbate chest pain.

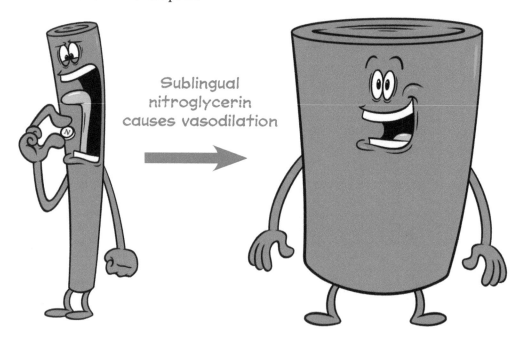

Sublingual nitroglycerin causes vasodilation

Cocaine

Cocaine use is associated with the development of acute myocardial ischemia and infarction. The incidence is much higher in young patients aged 18 to 45 years of age. Cocaine is a powerful sympathetic stimulator which causes an increase in heart rate, blood pressure, and myocardial contractility. Myocardial oxygen demand increases due to these processes. In addition, cocaine causes coronary artery vasoconstriction. The combination of excessive sympathetic stimulation and coronary artery vasoconstriction is a recipe for disaster that can lead to myocardial infarction.

Cocaine has also been shown to provoke a hypercoagulable state and cause acute thrombosis of the coronary arteries. Furthermore, cocaine may precipitate malignant ventricular arrhythmias in the setting of acute thrombosis and infarction. Cocaine exhibits class I and class III antiarrhythmic properties and prolongs the QT interval.

The ECG findings associated with cocaine use are not always indicative of ischemia or infarction, often demonstrating nonspecific ST segment and T wave changes. Troponin biomarkers are a sensitive and specific diagnostic tool for cocaine-induced MI. Cardiac observation is recommended when the diagnosis of cocaine-induced ACS is suspected but not immediately apparent.

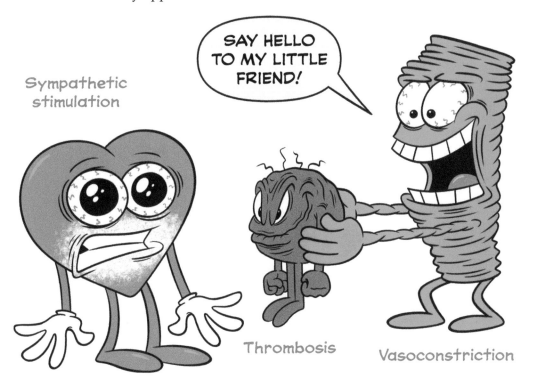

Pulmonary Embolism

The ECG manifestations of a pulmonary embolism (PE) include sinus tachycardia, incomplete or complete right bundle branch block, and nonspecific ST changes. PE is also associated with right axis deviation. In some cases the ECG may appear completely normal.

The S1Q3T3 pattern is commonly described as a classic ECG finding for PE, although it only occurs in about 15% of cases. The pattern consists of a S wave in lead I, a Q wave in lead III, and an inverted T wave in lead III.

Deep T wave inversions may appear in the anterior and inferior leads (II, III, aVF, V1-V4). It is important to keep PE at the top of your differential diagnosis list because this pattern may be mistaken for ACS.

A massive PE can cause acute cor pulmonale (right-sided heart failure) leading to dilation and ischemia of the right ventricle and dilation of the right atrium.

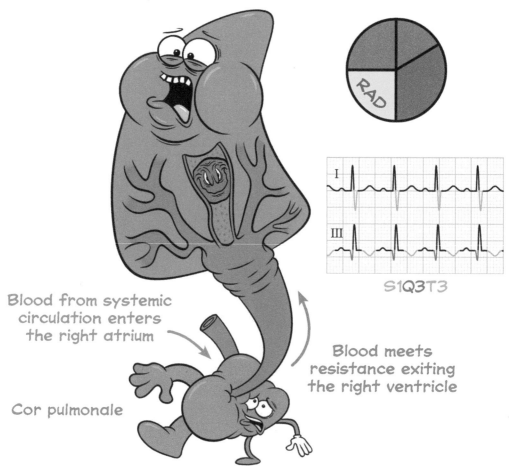

RAD

I

III

S1Q3T3

Blood from systemic circulation enters the right atrium

Blood meets resistance exiting the right ventricle

Cor pulmonale

Emphysema

The ECG of a patient with emphysema commonly demonstrates low voltage in the limb leads (i.e. the amplitude of the QRS complex is reduced). Low voltage is recorded because cardiac electrical activity is dampened by the large volume of trapped air in the lungs.

Other possible ECG findings include P pulmonale, right bundle branch block, and multifocal atrial tachycardia.

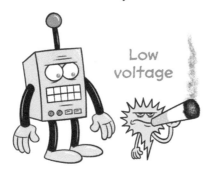

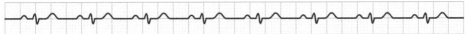

Emphysema causes pulmonary hypertension which leads to right ventricular hypertrophy and, eventually, cor pulmonale. Expansion of the lungs also compresses the heart into a more vertical position. These factors cause right axis deviation on the ECG.

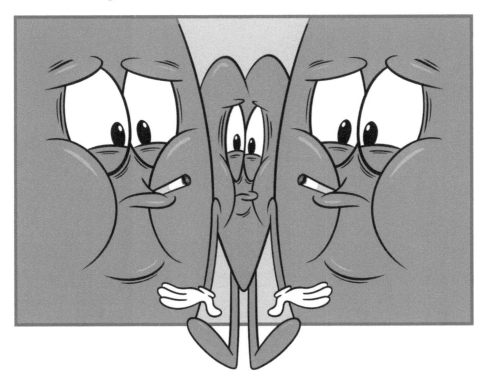

Hypothermia

Hypothermia is defined as a core body temperature less than 35°C (95°F). Such a low temperature slows electrical conduction and results in widening of the QRS complex with prolonged PR and QT intervals. Sinus bradycardia is common.

Hypothermia is frequently associated with the appearance of Osborn waves, which are also known as J waves because they occur at the J point. Osborn waves are characterized by a positive deflection at the end of the QRS complex. This type of ECG finding is also seen in a variety of other conditions including early repolarization and hypercalcemia. Very large and wide Osborn waves are more specific to hypothermia.

The ECG tracing may also demonstrate distortion (artifact) due to shivering from the patient. Moderate to severe hypothermia can lead to the development of atrial or ventricular fibrillation.

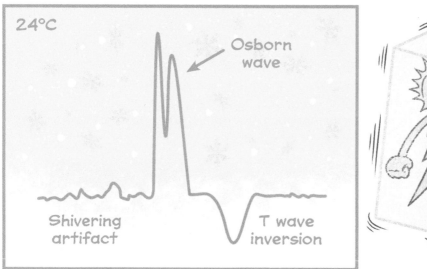

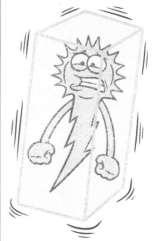

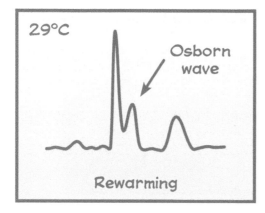

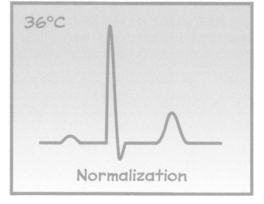

Raised Intracranial Pressure

ECG changes due to raised intracranial pressure are seen with subarachnoid hemorrhage (SAH), hemorrhagic stroke, traumatic brain injury, and other less common intracranial lesions.

The ECG pattern is characterized by giant T wave inversions, known as "cerebral T waves", and QT interval prolongation. An increase in U wave amplitude or bradycardia may also be seen.

The *Cushing reflex* is a physiological nervous system response to increased intracranial pressure that results in bradycardia, hypertension, and irregular breathing.

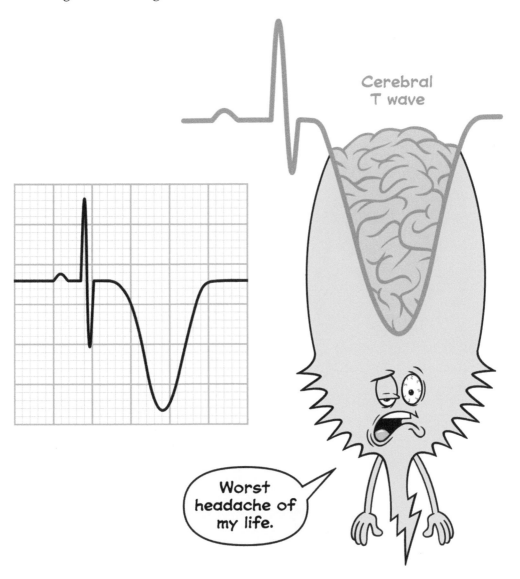

Pericardial Effusion

A pericardial effusion occurs when an excess amount of fluid accumulates in the fibroelastic sac surrounding the heart. If the pressure is great enough to impair diastolic filling and reduce cardiac output, then *cardiac tamponade* is considered to be present. Typical findings on the ECG include sinus tachycardia, low voltage, and electrical alternans.

In the context of a pericardial effusion, low voltage is attributed to the insulating effect of the fluid around the heart. Low voltage is defined as a QRS amplitude less than 5 mm in each of the limb leads and less than 10 mm in each of the precordial leads. Electrical alternans consists of beat-to-beat alternations in the height of the QRS complex caused by swinging of the heart in a large effusion.

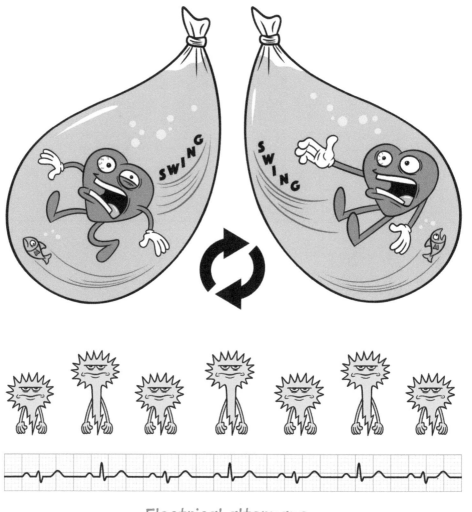

Electrical alternans

The Athlete's ECG

The ECG of an athlete commonly reflects benign changes that occur in the heart as a response to regular and sustained physical exercise. The heart undergoes structural and electrical remodeling which may mimic findings associated with pathologic heart processes, but these adaptations do not represent an increased risk of adverse events in asymptomatic athletes.

Possible findings in healthy athletes:

- Nonspecific ST segment elevation and T wave inversion
- First-degree or Mobitz type I (Wenckebach) AV block
- Sinus bradycardia ≥ 30 beats per minute
- Isolated QRS voltage criteria for LVH
- Junctional escape rhythm
- Ectopic atrial rhythm
- Incomplete RBBB

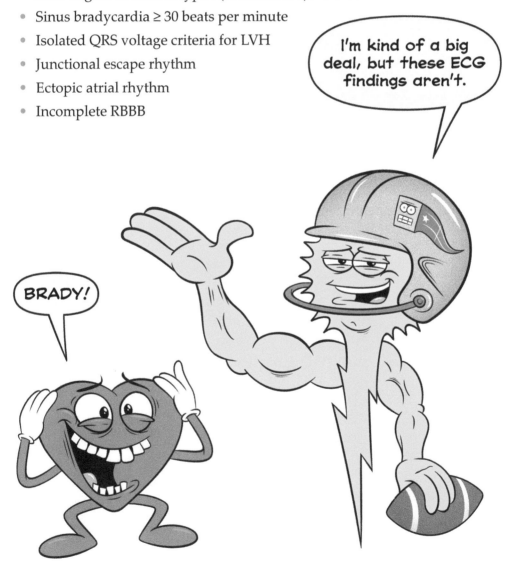

Hypertrophic Cardiomyopathy

Hypertrophic cardiomyopathy (HCM) is a genetic disorder characterized by diastolic dysfunction (impaired filling) due to thickening of the septum and left ventricle. This abnormal mass of cardiac muscle may block the left ventricular outflow tract (reducing cardiac output) and predispose the heart to the development of dangerous arrhythmias. Syncope, chest pain, dyspnea, palpitations, and ultimately, sudden death can result. HCM is the leading cause of sudden cardiac death among young athletes.

Treatment includes beta blockers or calcium channel blockers to improve diastolic dysfunction. Amiodarone may be used to treat ventricular arrhythmias. Symptoms that do not respond to medical management may require surgical intervention. ICD placement is considered in cases of HCM with syncope, sudden cardiac arrest, or confirmed ventricular arrhythmia.

ECG features of HCM:

- High voltage in the precordial leads
- Deep, narrow Q waves in the lateral and inferior leads - this finding is more common in the lateral leads than in the inferior leads
- Compensatory left atrial enlargement (P mitrale)
- Associated with Wolff-Parkinson-White syndrome

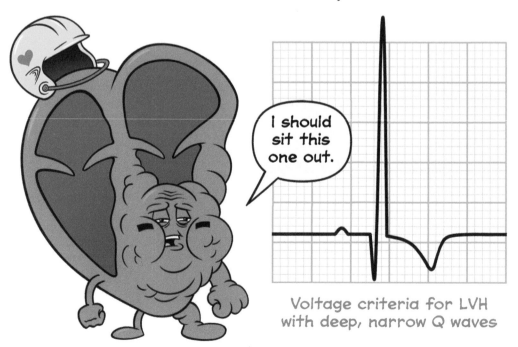

Voltage criteria for LVH with deep, narrow Q waves

Arrhythmogenic Right Ventricular Cardiomyopathy

Arrhythmogenic right ventricular cardiomyopathy (ARVC) is an important and under-recognized cause of sudden cardiac death in young adults and athletes. It is an inherited disorder characterized by atrophy of the ventricular wall and replacement with fibro-fatty tissue. The condition primarily affects the right ventricle but may also involve areas of the left ventricle.

Progression of the disease process leads to life-threatening ventricular arrhythmias and/or heart failure. Individuals with ARVC may be asymptomatic or present with palpitations, syncope, atypical chest pain, heart failure, or sudden cardiac death.

A characteristic ECG finding of ARVC is the *epsilon wave*. It is a small, distinct waveform occupying the initial part of the ST segment in the right precordial leads (V1 and V2).

ECG features of ARVC:

- Epsilon wave
- T wave inversion in V1-V3
- QRS complex widening
- Prolonged S wave upstroke ≥ 55 ms
- High incidence of PVCs and ventricular tachycardia

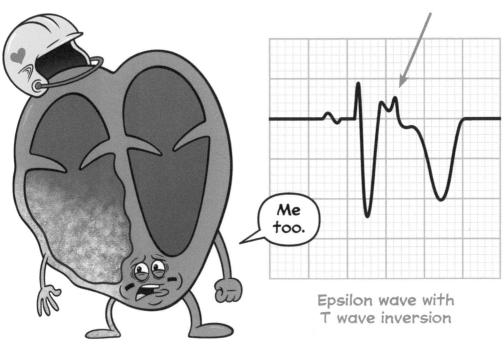

Epsilon wave with
T wave inversion

Concealed Conduction

Concealed conduction (CC) refers to electrical cardiac activity that is not directly visible on the ECG. The presence of an extra "hidden" impulse is deduced by analyzing the ECG for signs of its influence on subsequent electric impulses.

A nonrecordable electric impulse occurs when it partially travels through a part of the electrical conduction system without completing its full course. This impulse does not cause myocardial contraction, but it does result in electrophysiologic changes that affect the next impulse traveling by.

The manifestations of CC on the ECG include unexpected prolonged conduction, failure of impulse propagation, enhanced conduction, or pauses in the firing of a spontaneous pacemaker.

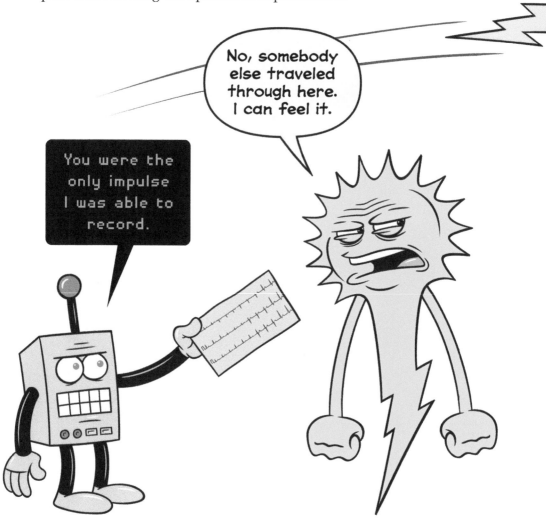

Sparkson's Summary: Chapter 10

- Hyperkalemia: serum potassium level greater than 5.0 mEq/L. ECG manifestations include peaked T waves, PR interval prolongation, QRS complex widening, and P wave flattening/disappearance.

- Hypokalemia: serum potassium level less than 3.5 mEq/L. ECG manifestations include ST depression, T wave flattening/inversion, and U wave development.

- Hypercalcemia: serum calcium level greater than 10.5 mg/dL, which causes a shortened QT interval.

- Hypocalcemia: serum calcium level less than 8.5 mg/dL, which causes a prolonged QT interval.

- Sodium channel blockers: slow conduction by inhibiting phase 0 of the action potential.

- Beta blockers: depress phase 4 of the pacemaker action potential and suppress sympathetic activity.

- Potassium channel blockers: lengthen the duration of phase 3 of the action potential, prolonging the refractory period.

- Non-dihydropyridine calcium channel blockers prolong conduction time and the refractory period in the AV node.

- Adenosine is an antiarrhythmic agent used to terminate supraventricular tachycardia involving the AV node.

- Digoxin increases vagal tone without decreasing contractility and has a narrow therapeutic range.

- Nitrates are used in the treatment of angina by causing vasodilation. They are contraindicated in the setting of RV infarction or with the use of phosphodiesterase-5 inhibitors.

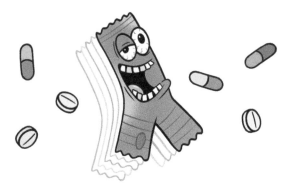

- Cocaine use is associated with acute myocardial infarction, especially in younger patients.

- Pulmonary embolism: ECG manifestations include sinus tachycardia, incomplete or complete RBBB, nonspecific ST changes, and the S1Q3T3 pattern.

- Emphysema: ECG findings include low voltage, P pulmonale, RBBB, and multifocal atrial tachycardia.

- Hypothermia: ECG findings include QRS complex widening, prolonged PR and QT intervals, and Osborn waves.

- Raised intracranial pressure: ECG findings include giant, inverted "cerebral" T waves and QT prolongation.

- A significant pericardial effusion or cardiac tamponade may manifest on the ECG with sinus tachycardia, low voltage, and electrical alternans.

- Healthy athletes may demonstrate a variety of benign ECG changes due to cardiac adaptations that occur with regular, sustained exercise.

- Hypertrophic cardiomyopathy (HCM): ECG findings include high voltage in the precordial leads and deep, narrow Q waves in the lateral and inferior leads.

- Arrhythmogenic right ventricular cardiomyopathy (ARVC): characteristic ECG finding is the epsilon wave.

- It is useful to obtain a prior ECG from the patient's records for comparison to determine if any new ECG findings are present.

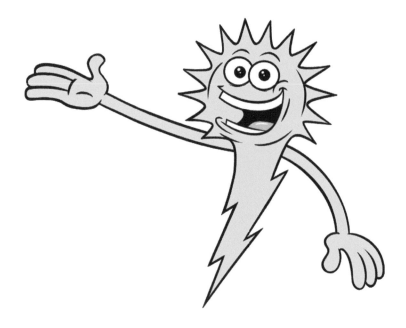

CHAPTER 11

CASE FILES

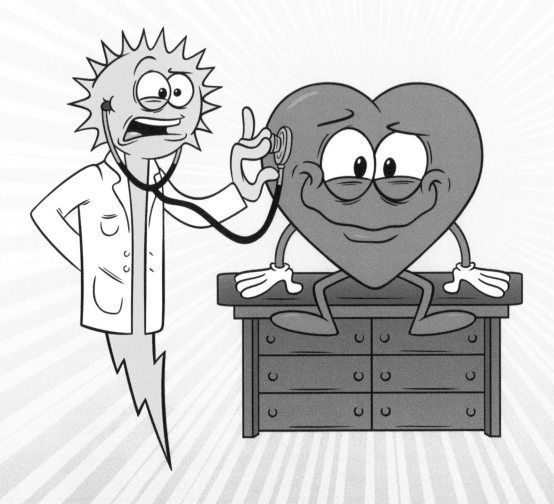

THIS section of the book will allow you to practice the art of ECG interpretation. The cases are presented with a brief history and an ECG tracing. Each ECG should be reviewed methodically to avoid missing important details. The following five-step approach is recommended when reviewing a 12-lead ECG:

1. *Calculate the rate.* The counting method is commonly used for regular heart rates. Search for an R wave that lands on a dark vertical line, and then use the subsequent dark line to begin counting off: **300, 150, 100, 75, 60, 50**. The 6-second method is useful for bradycardia and irregular rhythms. Count the number of QRS complexes within a 6 second interval and multiply that number by 10 for the estimated rate.

2. *Identify the underlying rhythm.* Assess the tracing for regularity and analyze the morphology of the waveforms. Check for normal P waves married with each QRS complex. Determine the duration of the QRS complex and the PR interval. Is there any evidence of preexcitation, AV block, bundle branch block, or fascicular block? Scan each lead and make note of abnormal waveforms, premature beats, pauses, or possible artifact.

3. *Determine the axis.* Feel free to use the rule of thumbs from chapter 5 as you focus your attention on leads I, aVF, and occasionally lead II.

4. *Check for hypertrophy and enlargement.* Do the P waves demonstrate evidence of atrial enlargement? Analyze leads V1, V5, and V6 for evidence of ventricular hypertrophy. Recognize repolarization abnormalities that may accompany ventricular hypertrophy.

5. *Examine for evidence of infarction.* Look for ST segment elevation or depression, pathologic Q waves, and T wave changes. If a STEMI is suspected, use lead groupings to determine the infarct location and likely culprit vessel. Recall your list of differential diagnoses and consider conditions that may mimic a STEMI.

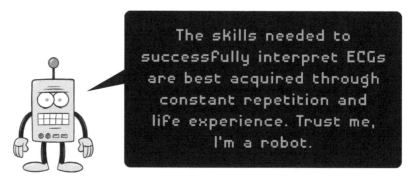

The skills needed to successfully interpret ECGs are best acquired through constant repetition and life experience. Trust me, I'm a robot.

CASE 1   29 year old asymptomatic male. He states he is an Olympic gold medalist and begins flexing his pecs.

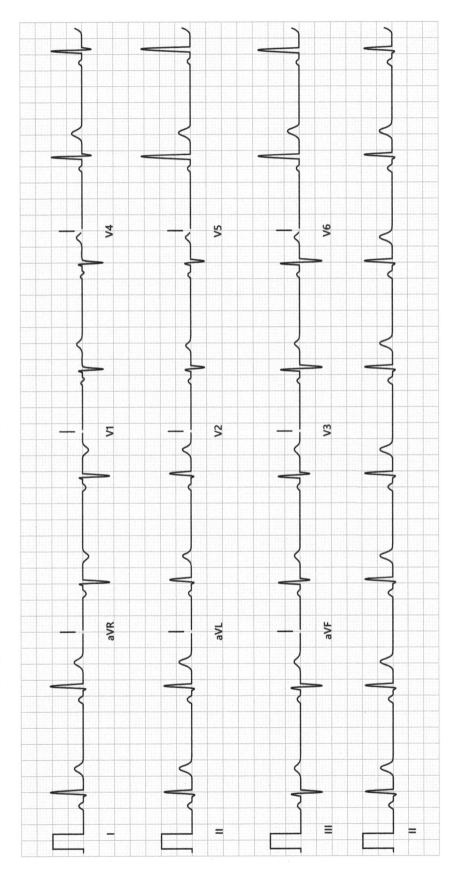

Case 1 Interpretation and Discussion

- Sinus bradycardia
- Rate around 43 BPM
- QRS interval less than 0.12 seconds
- Normal PR interval less than 0.2 seconds
- Normal axis

This patient has sinus bradycardia and is completely asymptomatic. Sinus bradycardia is defined as a heart rate less than 60 beats per minute. It is a common finding in healthy young adults and athletes, especially during sleep. Since this patient is asymptomatic, no treatment is necessary.

Sinus bradycardia can also be seen in healthy elderly patients, although this finding may represent an early manifestation of sinus node dysfunction. Other causes of sinus bradycardia include medications, myocardial infarction, hypothyroidism, vagal activation (e.g. carotid sinus stimulation, Valsalva maneuver, vomiting), increased intracranial pressure, and hypothermia among others.

Symptomatic sinus bradycardia should be treated according to the underlying condition. Atropine is typically utilized in cases of hemodynamic instability. When symptomatic bradycardia persists, the patient may require a permanent pacemaker.

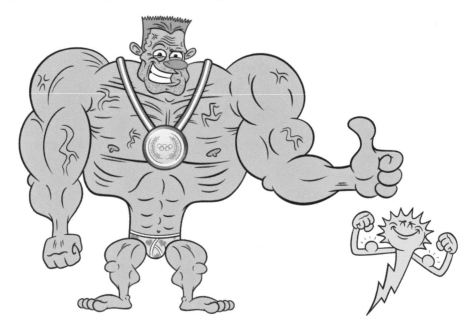

27 year old female complains of intermittent dizziness and palpitations. Her last episode occurred while surfing.

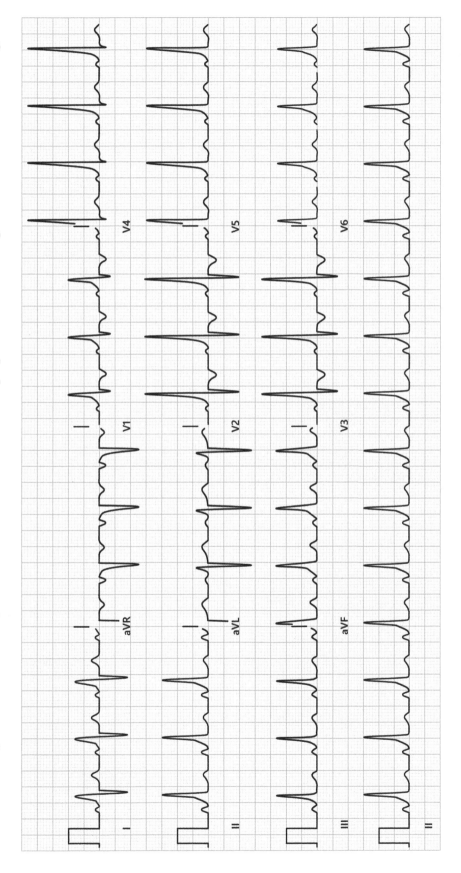

Case 2 Interpretation and Discussion

- Wolff-Parkinson-White syndrome
- Short PR interval less than 0.12 seconds
- Prolongation of the QRS interval greater than 0.11 seconds
- Delta wave: slurred upstroke of the QRS complex
- Prominent R waves in V1-V3 due to a left-sided accessory pathway

The WPW ECG pattern is characterized by a short PR interval followed by a delta wave. The majority of patients with this pattern remain asymptomatic. However, those with WPW *syndrome* have both the WPW pattern and episodes of paroxysmal tachyarrhythmias (e.g. AVRT). Patients that develop arrhythmias may experience symptoms such as palpitations, dizziness, syncope, or chest pain.

The accessory pathway, also known as the bundle of Kent, is a congenital bypass tract that can exist in a variety of locations within the heart. The majority of accessory pathways are located at the left free wall, and less commonly, in the posteroseptum, right free wall, or anteroseptum. An accessory pathway at the left free wall produces prominent R waves in V1, which can mimic posterior myocardial infarction or right bundle branch block. A large R wave in V1 is produced because a left sided pathway allows the impulse to bypass the AV node and travel through the myocardium from left to right.

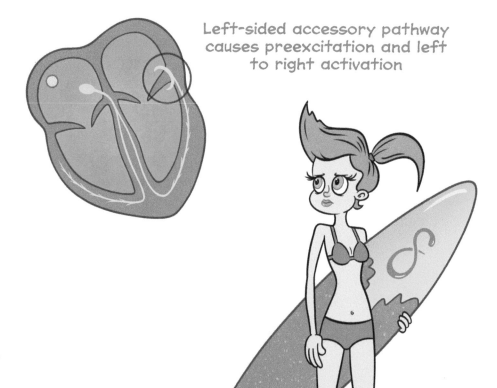

Left-sided accessory pathway causes preexcitation and left to right activation

CASE 3   70 year old male with hypertension. He admits to not taking his BP meds, but promises to start tomorrow.

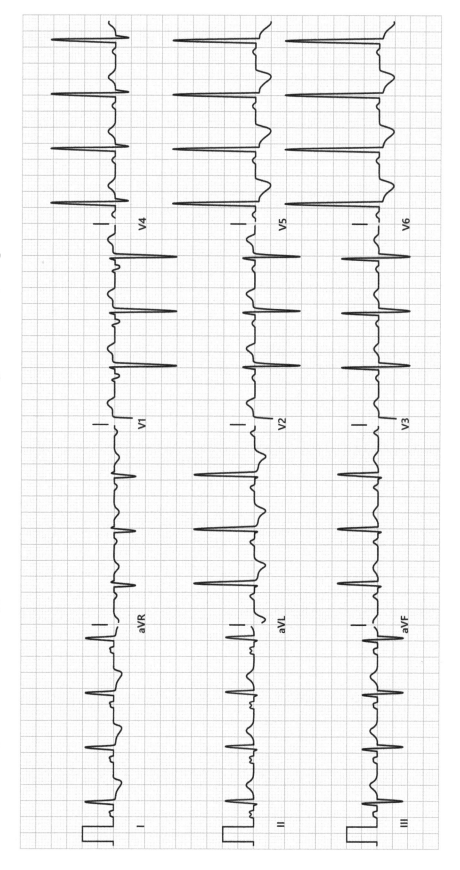

Case 3 Interpretation and Discussion

- Left ventricular hypertrophy
- Rate around 88 BPM
- Normal sinus rhythm
- P mitrale in leads II and V1
- T wave inversion in leads I, aVL, and V4-V6 (strain pattern)

LVH can occur in response to conditions that cause pressure or volume overload in the heart. Causes include systemic hypertension, aortic stenosis, aortic or mitral valve regurgitation, coarctation of the aorta, and hypertrophic cardiomyopathy.

Our patient in Case 3 has a long history of noncompliance with his blood pressure medications. LVH has developed in response to a state of chronic pressure overload. The *Sokolow-Lyon criteria* is most commonly used to determine LVH on the ECG:

- S wave in V1 + R wave in V5 or V6 > 35 mm
- R wave in aVL > 11 mm

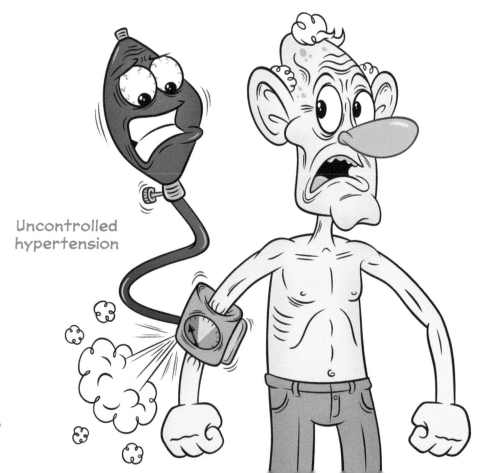

Uncontrolled hypertension

CASE 4 62 year old asymptomatic female presents complaining of a bad hare day.

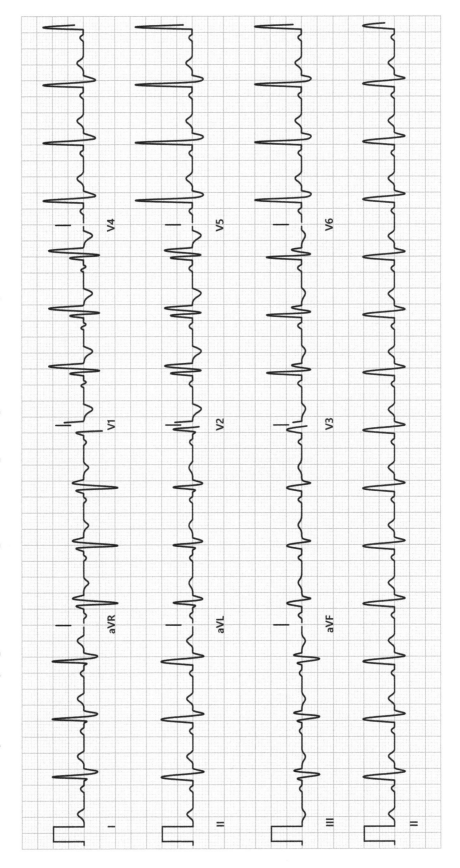

Case 4 Interpretation and Discussion

- Right bundle branch block
- Rate approximately 83 BPM
- QRS duration of 0.14 seconds
- Rabbit ears

    In the presence of a right bundle branch block, depolarization of the left ventricle proceeds normally while activation of the right ventricle is delayed. A prolonged QRS interval with characteristic morphological changes reflects the increase in time needed to depolarize the ventricles. In addition, leads V1-V3 may demonstrate ST segment depression and inverted T waves. The three major diagnostic criteria for RBBB are:

- QRS complex > 0.12 seconds
- RSR' pattern in leads V1 or V2
- Wide, slurred S waves in leads I and V6

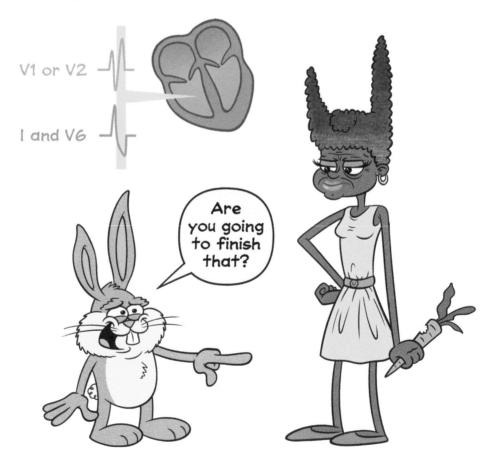

CASE 5 75 year old male with a history of type 2 diabetes and peripheral artery disease (PAD) complains of palpitations.

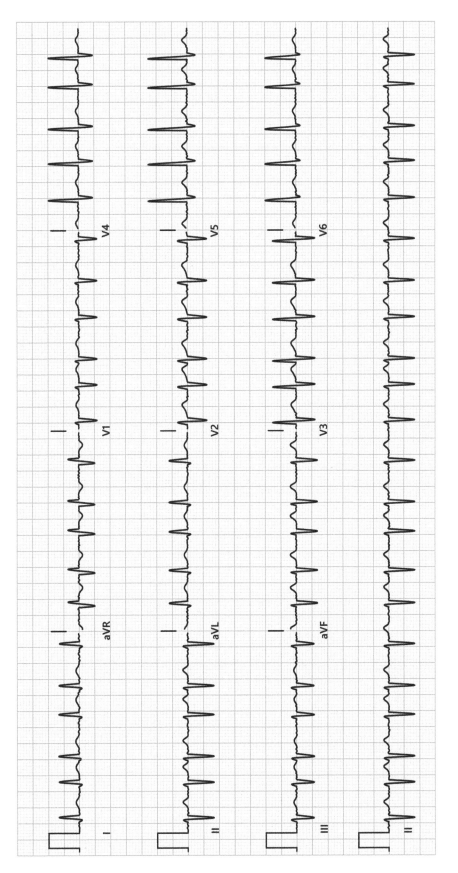

Case 5 Interpretation and Discussion

- Atrial fibrillation with rapid ventricular response
- Variable ventricular rate around 115 to 170 BPM
- Absence of discrete P waves
- Irregular rhythm
- Left axis deviation
- Left anterior fascicular block

Atrial fibrillation (AF) is the most common sustained arrhythmia. It is characterized on the ECG by an oscillating baseline of disorganized fibrillatory waves with an irregularly irregular ventricular response. The underlying mechanisms of AF are likely due to multiple wave reentry and/or focal firing from ectopic foci (most often in the pulmonary vein).

Possible symptoms related to AF include palpitations, fatigue, angina-like chest discomfort, dyspnea, and lightheadedness. Less frequently, syncope can occur due to a loss of the atrial kick and reduced cardiac output. It is also important to note that a significant minority of patients with AF have no symptoms at all.

AF is the most important cardiac cause of stroke. The atria quiver instead of contracting effectively, which promotes the blood stasis and thrombus formation. The source of embolic material is often suspected to be the left atrial appendage.

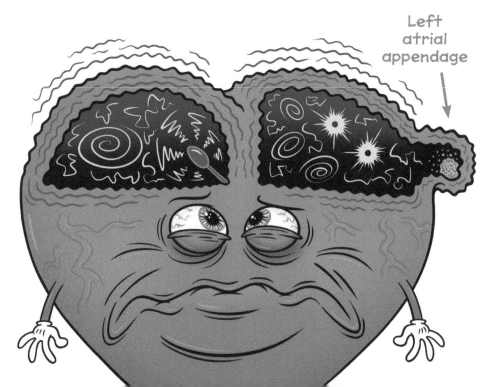

Left atrial appendage

Classification of atrial fibrillation:

- **Paroxysmal**: AF that terminates spontaneously or with intervention within 7 days of onset. Paroxysmal AF may occur episodically.

- **Persistent**: AF that is continuously present for greater than 7 days and up to 1 year.

- **Long-lasting persistent**: AF that has lasted more than 1 year with ongoing efforts to restore sinus rhythm.

- **Permanent**: AF that has continued for more than 1 year with failed efforts to restore and maintain sinus rhythm, and/or when rhythm control strategies are no longer sought.

Patients with AF at risk of stroke and systemic thromboemboli should receive anticoagulation therapy unless there is a specific contraindication. A useful tool to determine the level of stroke risk and aid in the selection of antithrombotic therapy is the *CHA_2DS_2-VASc index:

CHA_2DS_2-VASc risk criteria	Score
Congestive heart failure	1
Hypertension	1
Age 75 years or older	2
Diabetes mellitus	1
Stroke, TIA, or thromboembolism history	2
Vascular disease (PAD, prior MI, aortic plaque)	1
Age 65-74 years	1
Sex **C**ategory of female	1

The total score is used to guide treatment in nonvalvular AF. A score of 0 in males or 1 in females suggests a low risk of stroke and no antithrombotic therapy is recommended. A score of 1 in males suggests a moderate risk of stroke and aspirin or an oral anticoagulant is recommended. A score of 2 or more indicates a high risk of stroke and an oral anticoagulant is recommended. Patients with valvular heart disease accompanying their AF are also considered to be at high risk for an embolic event and are treated with anticoagulation.

* Pronounced "chads vasc."

AF can be caused by cardiovascular conditions including hypertension, coronary artery disease, myocardial infarction, heart failure, cardiomyopathy, valvular heart disease, pericardial disease, and disorders of the conduction system (e.g. WPW syndrome). AF can also be triggered by noncardiovascular conditions such as hyperthyroidism, sepsis, pulmonary disease, obstructive sleep apnea, and toxin exposure. Investigating all of these possibilities is important (e.g. obtaining an echocardiogram and thyroid function tests).

The management of AF is complex and varies depending on the patient's age, symptoms, hemodynamic status, comorbidities, underlying cause, and duration of AF. Management decisions that need to be addressed include the prevention of thromboembolism and a choice between a rate or rhythm control strategy.

Ventricular rate control is usually achieved with drugs such as beta blockers and non-dihydropyridine calcium channel blockers. In some cases AV node ablation with permanent pacemaker implantation may be indicated.

Strategies used to restore sinus rhythm include electrical cardioversion, antiarrhythmic drugs, and cardiac ablation. A common ablative technique involves electrically isolating the pulmonary veins to prevent the onset of AF. Restoring sinus rhythm does not eliminate the need for anticoagulation in patients at risk of stroke.

Some patients may benefit from a "pill in the pocket" approach to paroxysmal AF. This typically involves the self-administration of propafenone or flecainide at the onset of symptoms to restore sinus rhythm.

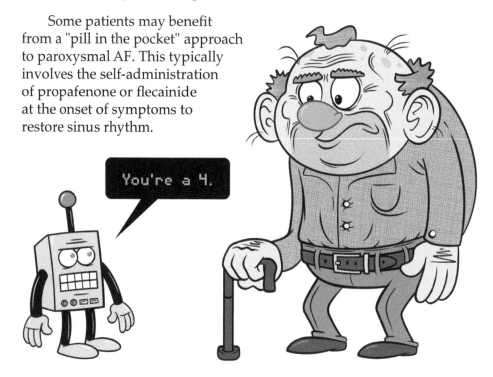

CASE 6   90 year old female calls 911 for acute chest pain and says, "Darlin', I have a sense of impending doom."

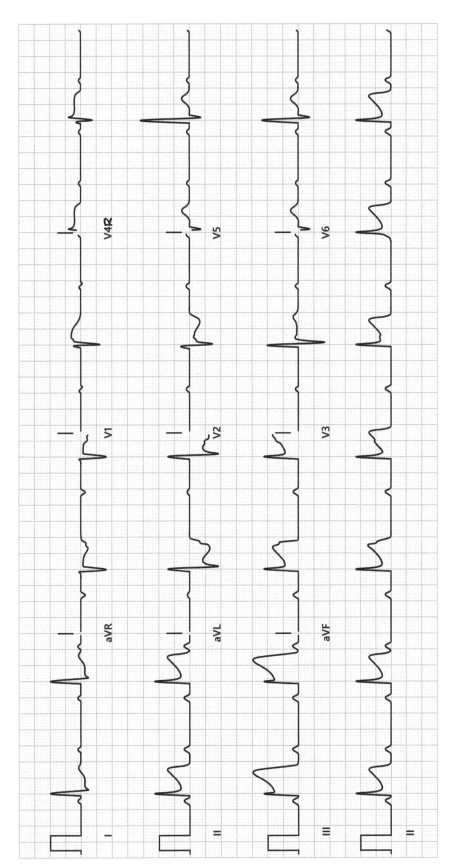

Case 6 Interpretation and Discussion

- Inferior STEMI with right ventricular infarction
- Atrial rate 94 BPM, ventricular rate 40 BPM
- Third degree AV block
- P waves and QRS complexes have no relation to each other
- Narrow QRS complex suggesting a junctional escape rhythm
- ST elevation in leads II, III, and AVF, with reciprocal ST depression in leads I and AVL
- ST elevation in the right-sided lead V4R

This ECG is highly suggestive of an occlusion of the proximal right coronary artery (RCA) with acute infarction of the inferior wall. ST elevation in lead III greater than in lead II and ST elevation in lead V1 indicate right ventricular involvement. A right sided lead was obtained to confirm the diagnosis. The AV node is also supplied by the RCA, and in this case AV nodal ischemia has resulted in complete heart block.

The patient's troponins were elevated and urgent echocardiography demonstrated a dilated right ventricle with hypokinesis, supporting the diagnosis of RV infarction. Nitrates negatively impact preload and are contraindicated in the setting of RV infarction. The patient was given IV fluids, aspirin, intravenous heparin, and statin therapy. Primary PCI was performed in less than 90 minutes.

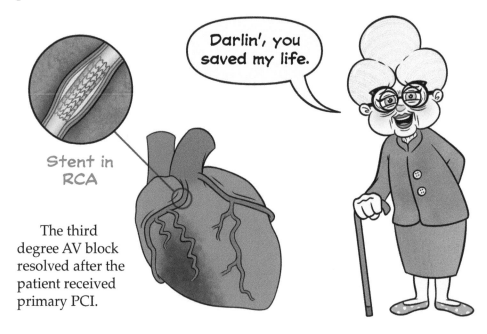

Stent in RCA

The third degree AV block resolved after the patient received primary PCI.

CASE 7   40 year old female complains of a sudden onset of palpitations and a feeling of "neck pounding."

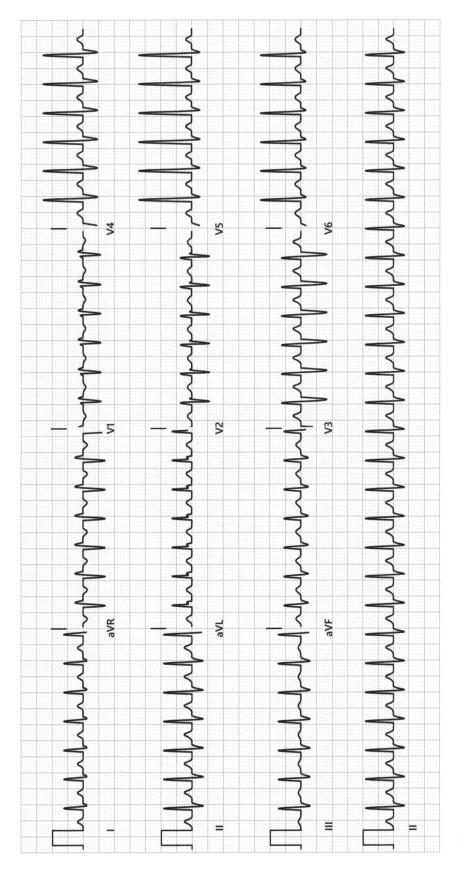

305

Case 7 Interpretation and Discussion

- AVNRT
- Rate 167 BPM
- Regular tachycardia
- No identifiable P waves
- Pseudo-R' wave in lead V1
- Notched QRS complex in lead aVL

The reentry circuit of AVNRT involves a slow and fast pathway into the AV node. The slow pathway conducts electric impulses at a relatively slow velocity, but recovers quickly from excitation (i.e. the slow pathway has a short refractory period). The fast pathway demonstrates a greater conduction velocity, but takes longer to recover from excitation (i.e. the fast pathway has a long refractory period).

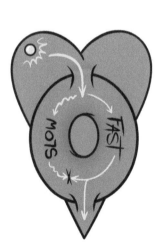 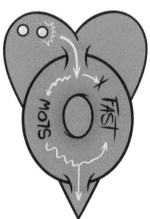 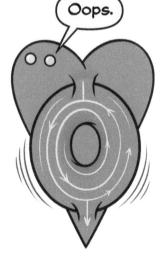

NSR: A regular impulse from the sinus node travels down the dual pathways. The slow impulse gets canceled out as the fast impulse is transmitted to the ventricles.

A PAC is blocked in the fast pathway due to the longer refractory period, conducts over the slow pathway, and travels retrograde up the now excitable fast pathway.

Typical (slow-fast) AVNRT ensues as the impulse is propagated through the reentry circuit in a continuous loop. Atypical variants of AVNRT are much less common.

AVNRT can be terminated by vagal maneuvers, adenosine, beta blockers, or non-dihydropyridine calcium channel blockers. Catheter ablation for AVNRT is highly effective for symptomatic patients.

CASE 8 54 year old male with chest pain and diaphoresis. After reviewing the ECG you develop diaphoresis as well.

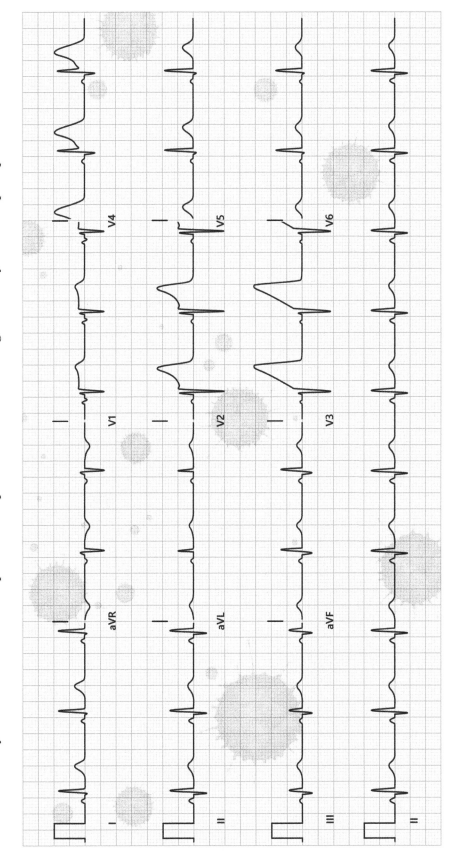

Case 8 Interpretation and Discussion

- Anteroseptal STEMI
- ST elevation in leads V1-V4
- Significant Q waves in leads II, III, and aVF
- Rate 60 BPM
- Sinus rhythm

The anteroseptal infarct pattern in this ECG is due to an acute occlusion of the LAD. Reciprocal changes are absent in this ECG because the infarct pattern did not involve the lateral wall. If the infarct extended laterally, there would likely be additional ST elevation in the lateral leads with reciprocal ST depression in the inferior leads. The Q waves in the inferior leads represent an age-indeterminate infarct. However, you were able to obtain a prior ECG from the patient's records and confirm that the Q waves in the inferior leads represent an old infarct. After wiping the sweat from your brow, you arrange for the patient to be transported to the cardiac cath lab.

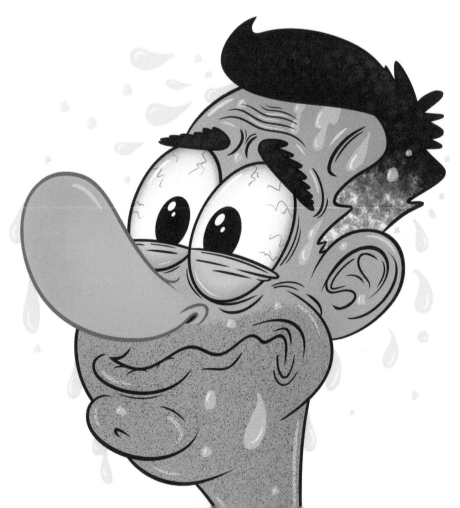

CASE 9 74 year old male with a history of syncope presents for a pacemaker check and complains of palpitations.

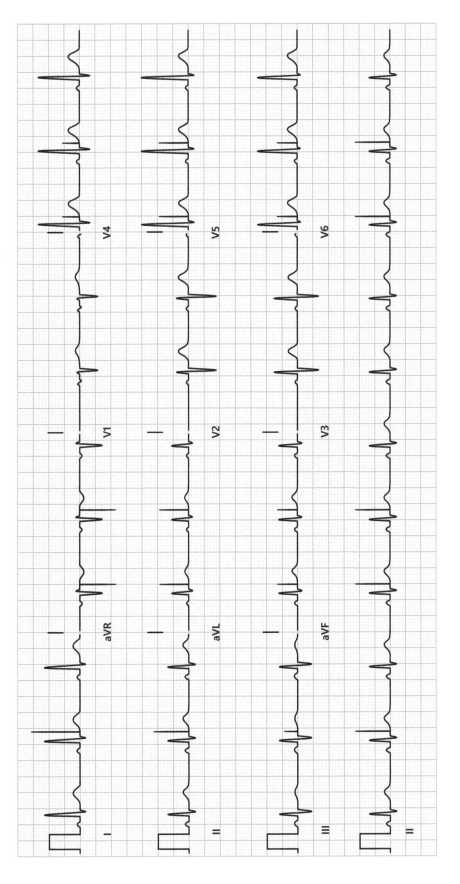

CASE 9 INTERPRETATION AND DISCUSSION

- Ventricular undersensing
- Inappropriately triggered pacing spikes
- Rate 65 BPM
- Normal sinus rhythm

This patient demonstrates a good intrinsic rhythm, but the pacemaker device fails to sense his native cardiac activity. Pacing spikes appear inappropriately after the QRS complex of the second, fourth, fifth, ninth, and tenth beats. The device has a sensing threshold that is too high relative to his native QRS complexes and requires reprogramming. Ventricular undersensing can be caused by lead wire displacement, lead wire fracture, improper sensing threshold, programming problems, or metabolic disturbances.

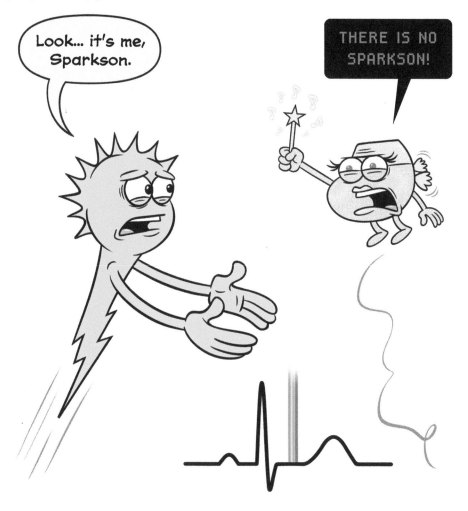

CASE 10   48 year old female with a history of schizophrenia follows up after being treated for pneumonia with azithromycin.

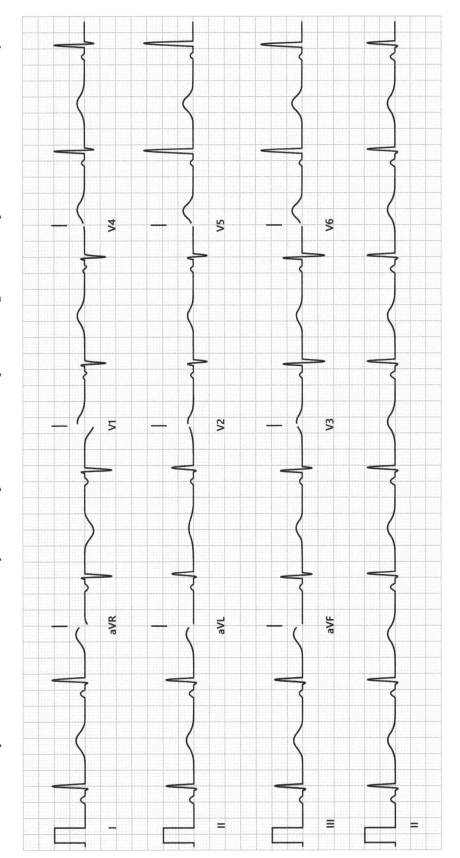

Case 10 Interpretation and Discussion

- QT prolongation
- Sinus bradycardia
- Normal QRS interval, PR interval, and axis
- QT interval of 0.88 seconds in lead II
- RR interval of 1.32 seconds
- *QTc of 0.765 seconds

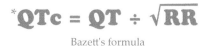

$$^*QTc = QT \div \sqrt{RR}$$

Bazett's formula

This patient has significant QT prolongation, which increases her risk of developing torsades de pointes. The patient's QT prolongation was acquired due to the concomitant use of antipsychotics and macrolide antibiotics. QT prolongation is also caused by electrolyte disturbances (e.g. hypokalemia, hypomagnesemia, hypocalcemia), or occur in the setting of acute myocardial infarction or stroke. QT prolongation may also be congenital in origin as seen in long QT syndrome (LQTS).

Drugs associated with QT prolongation

Antiarrhythmics	• Class IA: quinidine, procainamide, disopyramide • Class III: sotalol, dofetilide, ibutilide, amiodarone
Antipsychotics	• Haloperidol, chlorpromazine, droperidol, thioridazine, risperidone
Antidepressants	• Tricyclics: amitriptyline, desipramine • SSRIs: citalopram, fluoxetine
Antibiotics	• Fluoroquinolones: levofloxacin, ciprofloxacin, moxifloxacin • Macrolides: erythromycin, azithromycin
Others	• Methadone, antifungals, antiemetics

Note: this list is not comprehensive and does not reflect the risk of QT prolongation for each drug

CASE 11 52 year old male presents with chest pain and palpitations. He states he "doesn't feel so goo-" and passes out.

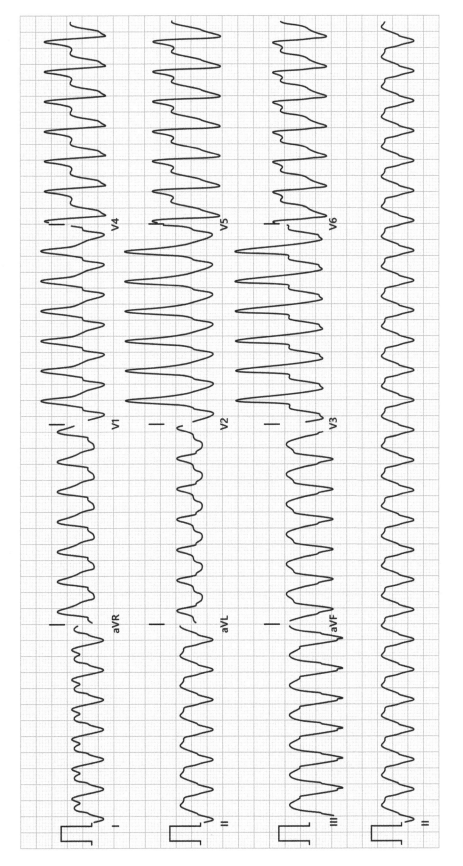

Case 11 Interpretation and Discussion

- Monomorphic ventricular tachycardia
- Rate around 170 BPM
- Regular rhythm
- Wide QRS complexes
- Extreme axis deviation

Unstable patients with sustained monomorphic VT require prompt treatment with synchronized electrical cardioversion. Hemodynamic instability may manifest as hypotension, altered mental status, chest pain, or heart failure. Management should proceed according to standard advanced cardiac life support (ACLS) resuscitation algorithms and any underlying causes for VT should be corrected. Stable patients with sustained VT may be treated with antiarrhythmic drug therapy such as IV lidocaine, procainamide, or amiodarone.

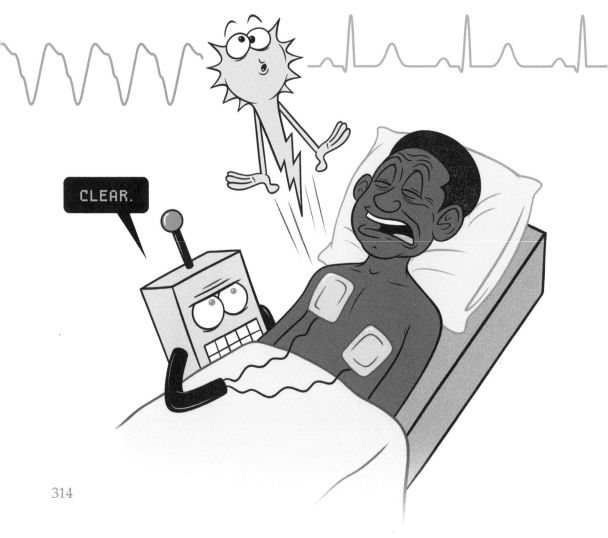

Quick Reference: Normal ECG Values

P wave

Duration: 0.06 - 0.12 seconds

Amplitude: Limb leads: less than 2.5 mm; precordial leads: less than 1.5 mm

Morphology: Upright in leads II and aVF; inverted in lead aVR; biphasic in lead V1

PR interval

Duration: 0.12 - 0.20 seconds

Morphology: Usually isoelectric. Depression of the PR segment less than 0.8 mm can be normal

QRS complex

Duration: 0.07 - 0.11 seconds

Amplitude: Limb leads: greater than 5 mm; R wave less than 11 mm in lead aVL; precordial leads: greater than 10 mm; R wave less than 18 mm in lead V6; high voltage may be a normal finding in young, athletic, or slim individuals

ST segment

Morphology: Usually isoelectric. ST segment can vary from 0.5 mm below to 1 mm above the baseline in limb leads, and up to 3 mm in the precordial leads (e.g. early repolarization)

T wave

Amplitude: Limb leads: less than 5 mm; precordial leads: less than 15 mm

QT interval

Duration: Upper limit of QTc is approximately 0.46 seconds

U wave

Morphology: Absent or present as a small wave following the T wave; deflection in same direction as the T wave

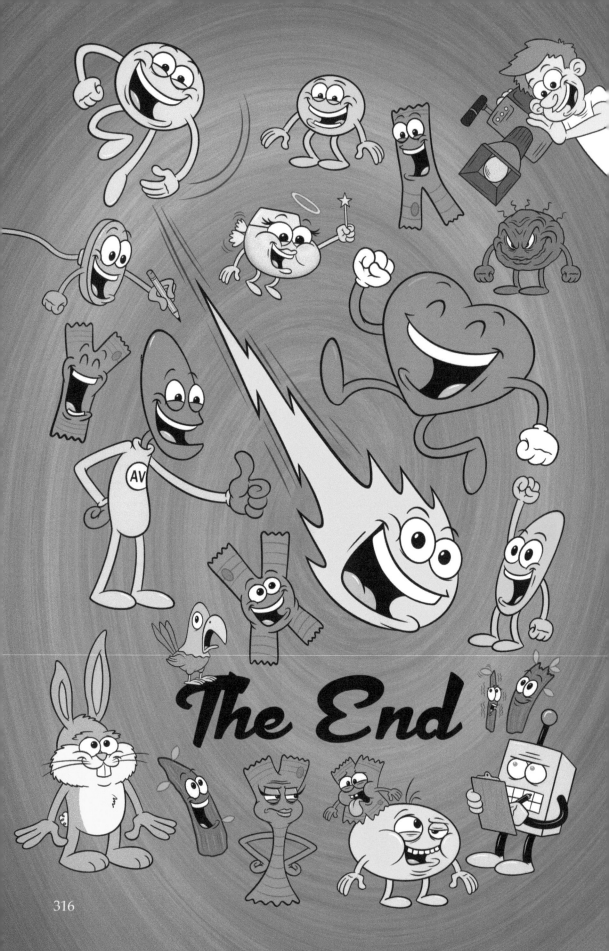

The End

About the Author

Jorge Muniz is the author and illustrator of *Medcomic: The Most Entertaining Way to Study Medicine* and *Sparkson's Illustrated Guide to ECG Interpretation*. He is a board certified PA from Orlando, Florida. He earned his Bachelor's degree in Biology in 2009 at George Mason University in Fairfax, Virginia. In 2013, he went on to complete his Master's degree in Medical Sciences at Nova Southeastern University (NSU) in Orlando, Florida.

Upon graduation from NSU, Jorge worked in the hospital setting in the field of orthopedic surgery. In 2015, he switched specialties to internal medicine, focusing on outpatient care. In 2018, Jorge embarked on a new journey to return to the hospital and become a cardiac electrophysiology PA.

Jorge has passions for art, education, entertainment, and medicine. His illustrations are influenced by old cartoons from his childhood. He is grateful for the opportunity to share these passions in a unique way and make a positive impact in communities around the world.

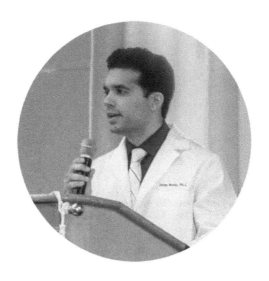

EPILOGUE: SELECTED REFERENCES

Chapter 1

Thomas, Stephen. "ECG File." Nursing Standard 4.29 (1990): 56-56.

Lux, Robert L. "Basis and ECG measurement of global ventricular repolarization." Journal of Electrocardiology 50.6 (2017): A1-A14.

Millar, Kay C. "Correlation between refractory periods and activation-recovery intervals from electrograms: effects of rate and adrenergic interventions." Circulation 72.6 (1985): 1372-1379.

Xie, Fagen, Zhilin Qu, Alan Garfinkel, and James N. Weiss. "Electrical refractory period restitution and spiral wave reentry in simulated cardiac tissue." AJP - Heart and Circulatory Physiology 283.1 (2002)H448.

Seigneuric, R.G., Chassé J.-L., P.M. Auger, and A.L. Bardou. "Role of the dispersion of refractoriness on cardiac reentries." Mathematical Biosciences 157.1 (1999): 253-267.

R. J. Myerburg, J. W. StewartS. M. Rossand B. F. Hoffman. "On-line measurement of duration of cardiac action potentials and refractory periods." Journal of Applied Physiology 28 (1970)92.

Trenor, Beatriz, Karen Cardona, Javier Saiz, Denis Noble, and Wayne Giles. "Cardiac action potential repolarization revisited: early repolarization shows all-or-none behaviour." The Journal of Physiology 595.21 (2017): 6599-6612.

Ho, Siew Yen, Robert H. Anderson, and Damián Sánchez-Quintana. "Atrial structure and fibres: morphologic bases of atrial conduction." Cardiovascular Research 54.2 (2002): 325-336.

Jacquemet, Vincent. "Modeling left and right atrial contributions to the ECG: A dipole-current source approach." Computers in Biology and Medicine 65 (2015): 192-199.

Tubbs, R. Shane, Robert H. Anderson, and Marios Loukas. "The anatomy of the cardiac conduction system." Clinical Anatomy 22.1 (2009): 99-113.

Wieling, Wouter, Frederik J. de Lange, and David L. Jardine. "The heart cannot pump blood that it does not receive." Frontiers in Physiology 5 (2014).

Felle, P., and J. G. Bannigan. "Anatomy of the valve of the coronary sinus (thebesian valve)." Clinical Anatomy 7.1 (1994): 10-12.

Navaratnam, V. "Design of heart valves: A review." Clinical Anatomy 6.6 (1993): 327-332.

Chapter 2

Bodin, O., D. Loginov, and N. Mitrokhina. "Improvement of ECG analysis for monitoring of cardiac electrical activity." Biomedical Engineering 42.3 (2008): 128-131.

Bagliani, G., F. Leonelli, L. Padeletti. "P Wave and the Substrates of Arrhythmias Originating in the Atria." Card Electrophysiol Clin. 9 (2017): 365-382. PubMed: 28838546.

Soto-Bernal, J. J., J. Mascorro-Pantoja, and G. A. Pérez-Herrera. "Heart activity monitoring using a Michelson interferometer." Proceedings of SPIE 6046.1 (2006): 604603-604603-6.

Rajendra Acharya, U., P. Subbanna Bhat, and U.C. Niranjan. "Comprehensive visualization of cardiac health using electrocardiograms." Computers in Biology and Medicine 32.1 (2002): 49-54.

Bhaskar, Anand, and Arati Vinod. "Demonstration of the Origin of ECG Waves." Advances in Physiology Education 30.3 (2006)128.

Magnani, Jared W. "Risk assessment for atrial fibrillation: Enter the P-wave." Heart Rhythm 12.9 (2015): 1896-1897.

Ishida, Katsuya, Hideki Hayashi, Akashi Miyamoto, Yoshihisa Sugimoto, Makoto Ito, Yoshitaka Murakami, and Minoru Horie. "P wave and the development of atrial fibrillation." Heart Rhythm 7.3 (2010): 289-294.

de Luna, Antoni Bayes. "Evolution of electrocardiographic terminology for walls of the heart and "Q-wave" myocardial infarction." Journal of Electrocardiology 41.5 (2008): 423-424.

Bogossian, Harilaos, Ilias Ninios, Gerrit Frommeyer, Dejan Mijic, Fuad Hasan, Dirk Bandorski, Lars Eckardt, Bernd Lemke, and Markus Zarse. "Q Wave in the Inferior Leads: There Is More Than Scar." Annals of Noninvasive Electrocardiology 20.6 (2015): 609-611.

Poole, Jeanne E., Jagmeet P. Singh, and Ulrika Birgersdotter-Green. "QRS Duration or QRS Morphology." Journal of the American College of Cardiology 67.9 (2016): 1104-1117.

Meyerowitz, Eric A., and Ralph J. Verdino. "The case of a missing QRS complex." Journal of Electrocardiology 48.5 (2015): 907-908.

Sharma, Tanushree, and Kamalesh Kumar Sharma. "QRS complex detection in ECG signals using locally adaptive weighted total variation denoising." Computers in Biology and Medicine 87 (2017): 187-199.

Oosterom, Aadiaan van. "The Dominant T Wave and Its Significance." Journal of Cardiovascular Electrophysiology 14 (2003): S180-S187.

Meijborg, V.M.F., C.N.W. Belterman, J.M.T. de Bakker, R. Coronel, and C.E. Conrath. "Mechano-electric coupling, heterogeneity in repolarization and the electrocardiographic T-wave." Progress in Biophysics & Molecular Biology 130 (2017): 356-364.

Kukla, Piotr, Adrian Baranchuk, Marek Jastrzębski, and Leszek Bryniarski. "U Wave Variability in the Surface ECG." Annals of Noninvasive Electrocardiology 19.6 (2014): 601-603.

Eyer, Kenneth. "Support for a mechanico-electrical source of the "U" wave." Journal of Electrocardiology 48.1 (2015): 31-32.

Houssein, Essam H., Moataz Kilany, and Aboul Ella Hassanien. "ECG signals classification: a review." International Journal of Intelligent Engineering Informatics 5.4 (2017): 376-396.

Chen, Xu-Miao, Cheng-Cheng Ji, Yun-Jiu Cheng, Li-juan Liu, Wei-Qi Zhu, Ying Huang, Wei-Ying Chen, and Su-Hua Wu. "The Role of the Ratio of J-Point Elevation Magnitude and R-Wave Amplitude on the Same ECG Lead in the Risk Stratification of Subjects With Early Repolarization Pattern." Clinical Cardiology 39.11 (2016): 678-683.

Maeda, Toshihiro, Tetsunori Saikawa, Hiroko Niwa, Nobuo Shimoyama, Masahide Hara, Tohru Maruyama, Ryosaburo Takaki, Morio Ito, and Kohsei Kohmatsu. "QT interval shortening and ST elevation in intracoronary ECG during PTCA." Clinical Cardiology 15.7 (1992): 525-528.

Batchvarov, Velislav N., Azad Ghuran, Peter Smetana, Katerina Hnatkova, Monica Harries, Polychronis Dilaveris, A. John Camm, and Marek Malik. "QT-RR relationship in healthy subjects exhibits substantial intersubject variability and high intrasubject stability." AJP - Heart and Circulatory Physiology 282.6 (2002)H2356.

Brouwer, Jan, Maarten P. Van Den Berg, Diederick E. Grobbee, Jaap Haaksma, and Arthur A.M. Wilde. "Diagnostic Performance of Various QTc Interval Formulas in a Large Family with Long QT Syndrome Type 3: Bazett's Formula Not So Bad After All …." Annals of Noninvasive Electrocardiology 8.4 (2003).

Pasquier, M., O. Pantet, O. Hugli, E. Pruvot, T. Buclin, G. Waeber, and D. Aujesky. "Prevalence and determinants of QT interval prolongation in medical inpatients." Internal Medicine Journal 42.8 (2012).

Chapter 3

Dohare, A., V. Kumar, and R. Kumar. "12-lead ECG analysis based on composite lead signal." Journal of Electrocardiology 46.4 (2013): e30-e31.

Alinier, Guillaume, Ray Gordon, Colin Harwood, and William B Hunt. "12-Lead ECG training: The way forward." Nurse Education Today 26.1 (2006): 87-92.

Drew, Barbara, and Paul Kligfield. "Standardizing electrocardiographic leads: introduction to a symposium." Journal of Electrocardiology 41.3 (2008): 187-189.

Kennedy, Alan, Dewar D. Finlay, Daniel Guldenring, Raymond R. Bond, David J. McEneaney, Aaron Peace, and James McLaughlin. "Improved recording of atrial activity by modified bipolar leads derived from the 12-lead electrocardiogram." Journal of Electrocardiology 48.6 (2015): 1017-1021.

Benjamin E. Jin, Heike WulffJonathan H. WiddicombeJie ZhengDonald M. Bersand Jose L. Puglisi. "A simple device to illustrate the Einthoven triangle." Advances in Physiology Education 36.4 (2012)319.

Riera, Andrés Ricardo Pérez, Celso Ferreira, Celso Ferreira Filho, Sergio Dubner, Raimundo Barbosa Barros, Francisco Femenía, and Adrian Baranchuk. "Clinical Value of Lead aVR." Annals of Noninvasive Electrocardiology 16.3 (2011).

Pahlm, Olle, and Galen S. Wagner. "Potential solutions for providing standard electrocardiogram recordings from nonstandard recording sites." Journal of Electrocardiology 41.3 (2008): 207-210.

Kania, Michał, Hervé Rix, Małgorzata Fereniec, Heriberto Zavala-Fernandez, Dariusz Janusek, Tomasz Mroczka, Günter Stix, and Roman Maniewski. "The effect of precordial lead displacement on ECG morphology." Medical & Biological Engineering & Computing 52.2 (2013): 109-119.

Gregg, Richard E., Sophia H. Zhou, James M. Lindauer, Dirk Q. Feild, and Eric D. Helfenbein. "Where do derived precordial leads fail?." Journal of Electrocardiology 41.6 (2008): 546-552.

Zywietz, C., D. Celikag, and G. Joseph. "Influence of ECG measurement accuracy on ECG diagnostic statements." Journal of Electrocardiology 29 (1996): 67-72.

Chapter 4

Mont, Lluís. "'Fight for sinus rhythm, or surrender?'...." European Heart Journal 35.22 (2014): 1427-1429.

Schuessler, Richard B., John P. Boineau, and Burt I. Bromberg. "Origin of the Sinus Impulse." Journal of Cardiovascular Electrophysiology 7.3 (1996).

Coumel, Philippe. "Cardiac Arrhythmias and the Autonomic Nervous System." Journal of Cardiovascular Electrophysiology 4.3 (1993).

Luft, Caroline Di Bernardi, Emílio Takase, and David Darby. "Heart rate variability and cognitive function: Effects of physical effort." Biological Psychology 82.2 (2009): 186-191.

Attias, Julia, Julie Bieles, Philip Carvil, Charles Laing, Fiona Lewis, Oihane Jaka, Katie O'Brien, and Prashant Ruchaya. "Altitude exposure and increased heart rate: the role of the parasympathetic nervous system." The Journal of Physiology 595.14 (2017): 4589-4590.

Kearney, Kathleen, Sonja Ellingson, Karen Stout, and Kristen K. Patton. "From Bradycardia to Tachycardia: Complete Heart Block." The American Journal of Medicine 128.7 (2015): 702-706.

Handa, Kushal, Anita Arnold, Zalmen Blanck, Masood Akhtar, and Mohammad-Reza Jazayeri. "Syncope in the Presence of Newly Developed Bundle Branch Block: Bradycardia or Tachycardia Related." Pacing and Clinical Electrophysiology 20.10 (1997).

Hall, Kevin, and Leon Glass. "Locating Ectopic Foci." Journal of Cardiovascular Electrophysiology 10.3 (1999).

Garson, Arthur, Paul C. Gillette, Jeffrey P. Moak, James C. Perry, David A. Ott, and Denton A. Cooley. "Supraventricular Tachycardia Due to Multiple Atrial Ectopic Foci: A Relatively Common Problem." Journal of Cardiovascular Electrophysiology 1.2 (1990).

Saint, David A. "Pacemaking in the Heart: The Interplay of Ionic Currents." Clinical and Experimental Pharmacology and Physiology 25.10 (1998).

Hsieh, Ming-Hsiung, Ching-Tai Tai, Chin-Feng Tsai, Wen-Chung Yu, Wei-Shiang Lin, Jin-Long Huang, Yu-An Ding, Mau-Song Chang, and Shih-Ann Chen. "Mechanism of Spontaneous Transition from Typical Atrial Flutter to Atrial Fibrillation: Role of Ectopic Atrial Fibrillation Foci." Pacing and Clinical Electrophysiology 24.1 (2001).

Fleisher, Lee A. "Heart rate variability as an assessment of cardiovascular status." Journal of Cardiothoracic and Vascular Anesthesia 10.5 (1996): 659-671.

Birand, Ahmet, Sokol Saliu, and Gulmira Z. Kudaiberdieva. "Time-Frequency Analysis of Heart Rate Variability." Annals of Noninvasive Electrocardiology 1.4 (1996).

Rabiner, Joni E., Michele J. Fagan, and Christine A. Walsh. "Can You Read This Electrocardiogram?." Clinical Pediatric Emergency Medicine 12.4 (2011): 333-342.

Massin, M., and G. von Bernuth. "Normal Ranges of Heart Rate Variability During Infancy and Childhood." Pediatric Cardiology 18.4 (2014): 297-302.

Sottas, Cedric E., David Cumin, Brian J. Anderson, and Laszlo Vutskits. "Blood pressure and heart rates in neonates and preschool children: an analysis from 10 years of electronic recording." Pediatric Anesthesia 26.11 (2016): 1064-1070.

Hussein, Ahmed, Shaiful Hashim, Ahmad Aziz, Fakhrul Rokhani, and Wan Adnan. "Performance Evaluation of Time-Frequency Distributions for ECG Signal Analysis." Journal of Medical Systems 42.1 (2017): 1-16.

Chapter 5

Bacharova, Ljuba. "Changing role of ECG in the evaluation left ventricular hypertrophy." Journal of Electrocardiology 45.6 (2012): 609-611.

Ip, James E. "Localization of ventricular arrhythmias: The importance of evaluating the frontal axis." Journal of Cardiovascular Electrophysiology 28.10 (2017): 1187-1188.

Spodick, David H., Mary Frisella, and Sirin Apiyassawat. "QRS Axis Validation in Clinical Electrocardiography." The American Journal of Cardiology 101.2 (2008): 268-269.

Macfarlane, Peter W. "The frontal plane QRS-T angle." Europace 14.6 (2012): 773-775.

Yochai, Birnbaum. "About QRS prolongation, distortion and the acuteness score." Journal of Electrocardiology 49.3 (2016): 265-271.

Barold, S. Serge. "Reappraisal of ECG Lead V1 in the Assessment of Cardiac Resynchronization." Pacing and Clinical Electrophysiology 38.3 (2015): 291-294.

Pantazopoulos, John, Alice David, Nora M. Cosgrove, and John B. Kostis. "Left Axis Deviation as a Risk Marker in Patients Without Ischemic Heart Disease." Journal of the American College of Cardiology 67.13 (2016).

Nikolic, George. "Left bundle branch block with right axis deviation." Heart & Lung: The Journal of Acute and Critical Care 24.4 (1995): 345-346.

Spodick, David H., Mary Frisella, and Sirin Apiyassawat. "QRS Axis Validation in Clinical Electrocardiography." The American Journal of Cardiology 101.2 (2008): 268-269.

Mori, Shumpei, Robert H Anderson, Natsuko Tahara, Yu Izawa, Takayoshi Toba, Sei Fujiwara, Shinsuke Shimoyama, Yoshiaki Watanabe, Tatsuya Nishii, Atsushi K Kono, and Ken-Ichi Hirata. "Diversity and Determinants of the Three-dimensional Anatomical Axis of the Heart as Revealed Using Multidetector-row Computed Tomography." The Anatomical Record : Advances in Integrative Anatomy and Evolutionary Biology 300.6 (2017): 1083-1092.

Wilde, A. "An atypical arrhythmia." Netherlands Heart Journal 21.5 (2013): 262-262.

Chapter 6

Biolato, Marco, Massimo Montalto, Alfonso Sestito, Antonella Gallo, and Antonio Grieco. "ECG signs of biatrial enlargement in a young adult." Internal and Emergency Medicine 5.5 (2010): 441-442.

Katz, Arnold M. "Evolving concepts of heart failure: Cooling furnace, malfunctioning pump, enlarging muscle: Part II: Hypertrophy and dilatation of the failing heart." Journal of Cardiac Failure 4.1 (1998): 67-81.

Peenen, Hubert J., and Bruno Gerstl. "Arteriosclerotic Massive Hypertrophy of the Heart." Journal of American Geriatrics Society 10.6 (1962).

Su, Guanhua, Heng Cao, Sudan Xu, Yongxin Lu, Xinxin Shuai, Yufei Sun, Yuhua Liao, and Jingdong Li. "Left Atrial Enlargement in the Early Stage of Hypertensive Heart Disease: A Common But Ignored Condition." Journal of Clinical Hypertension 16.3 (2014): 192-197

Pelliccia, Antonio, Martin S. Maron, and Barry J. Maron. "Assessment of Left Ventricular Hypertrophy in a Trained Athlete: Differential Diagnosis of Physiologic Athlete's Heart From Pathologic Hypertrophy." Progress in Cardiovascular Diseases 54.5 (2012): 387-396.

Verdecchia, Paolo, Fabio Angeli, Giovanni Mazzotta, Giuseppe Ambrosio, and Gianpaolo Reboldi. "Simplifying the ECG Diagnosis of Left Ventricular Hypertrophy." Current Cardiovascular Risk Reports 5.1 (2010): 1-4.

Estes, E. Harvey. "ECG manifestations of left ventricular electrical remodeling." Journal of Electrocardiology 45.6 (2012): 612-616.

Barold, S. Serge, and Ary L. Goldberger. "A Specific ECG Triad Associated with Congestive Heart Failure." Pacing and Clinical Electrophysiology 5.4 (1982).

Ishida, Katsuya, Hideki Hayashi, Akashi Miyamoto, Yoshihisa Sugimoto, Makoto Ito, Yoshitaka Murakami, and Minoru Horie. "P wave and the development of atrial fibrillation." Heart Rhythm 7.3 (2010): 289-294.

Akiyama, Toshio, and James P. Eichelberger. "Interatrial block vs left atrial enlargement." Journal of Electrocardiology 45.5 (2012): 452-453.

Pia, MariaCalabrò, Giuseppe Oreto, and Salvatore Consolo. "Post-ventricular tachycardia p wave change simulating atrial enlargement." Journal of Electrocardiology 31.1 (1998): 67-70.

Xiao, HB., S. Rizvi, D. Mccrea, B. Kaufman, and M. Dancy. "Right Atrial Enlargement in Atrial Fibrillation." Age and Ageing 27.suppl_2 (1998): 21-c-22.

Allison, John D., Francisco Yuri Macedo, Ihab Rafic Hamzeh, and Yochai Birnbaum. "Correlation of right atrial enlargement on ECG to right atrial volume by echocardiography in patients with pulmonary hypertension." Journal of Electrocardiology 50.5 (2017): 555-560.

Levin, Aaron R., Mira Frand, and Harold A. Baltaxe. "Left Atrial Enlargement." Radiology 104.3 (1972)615.

Bacharova, Ljuba. "The 1st symposium on ECG changes in left or right ventricular hypertension or hypertrophy in conditions of pressure overload." Journal of Electrocardiology 47.5 (2014): 589-592.

Chapter 7

Katritsis, Demosthenes G., George C.M. Siontis, and A. John Camm. "Prognostic Significance of Ambulatory ECG Monitoring for Ventricular Arrhythmias." Progress in Cardiovascular Diseases 56.2 (2013): 133-142.

Luz, Eduardo José da S., Thiago M. Nunes, Victor Hugo C. de Albuquerque, João P. Papa, and David Menotti. "ECG arrhythmia classification based on optimum-path forest." Expert Systems with Applications 40.9 (2013): 3561-3573.

Poulikakos, Dimitrios, and Marek Malik. "Challenges of ECG monitoring and ECG interpretation in dialysis units." Journal of Electrocardiology 49.6 (2016): A1-A10.

Subbiah, Rajeeve, and Pravin Patil. "Arrhythmias in vasodilator stress testing." Journal of Nuclear Cardiology 24.2 (2016): 410-412.

Drouin, Emmanuel. "Electrophysiologic Properties of the Adult Human Sinus Node." Journal of Cardiovascular Electrophysiology 8.3 (1997).

Lüscher, Thomas F. "Supraventricular and ventricular arrhythmias." European Heart Journal 36.46 (2015): 3215-3217.

"Supraventricular arrhythmias in the elderly: choose therapy with care." Drugs & Therapy Perspectives 11.7 (2012): 5-8.

Wellens, Hein J.J. "Twenty-Five Years of Insights into the Mechanisms of Supraventricular Arrhythmias." Journal of Cardiovascular Electrophysiology 14.9 (2003).

Padmanabhan, Deepak, Alan Sugrue, Prakriti Gaba, and Samuel Asirvatham. "Outflow tract ventricular arrhythmias." Herzschrittmachertherapie + Elektrophysiologie 28.2 (2017): 177-186.

Batra, Anjan, and Michael J. Silka. "Ventricular arrhythmias." Progress in Pediatric Cardiology 11.1 (2000): 39-45.

Hetland, Mathias, Kristina H. Haugaa, Sebastian I. Sarvari, Gunnar Erikssen, Erik Kongsgaard, and Thor Edvardsen. "A Novel ECG-Index for Prediction of Ventricular Arrhythmias in Patients after Myocardial Infarction." Annals of Noninvasive Electrocardiology 19.4 (2014): 330-337.

Patel, S. "Sinus arrest on the electrocardiograph: pseudo or real?." Acta Anaesthesiologica Scandinavica 53.6 (2009).

Katoh, Takakazu, and Shinji Kinoshita. "Mechanism of atrial escape-capture bigeminy: Second-degree sinoatrial exit and entrance block." Journal of Electrocardiology 31.2 (1998): 145-149.

Jensen, Paul N., Noelle N. Gronroos, Lin Y. Chen, Aaron R. Folsom, Chris deFilippi, Susan R. Heckbert, and Alvaro Alonso. "Incidence of and Risk Factors for Sick Sinus Syndrome in the General Population. Rajawat, Yadavendra S., Edward P. Gerstenfeld, Vickas V. Patel, Sanjay Dixit, David J. Callans, and Francis E. Marchlinski. "ECG Criteria for Localizing the Pulmonary Vein Origin of Spontaneous Atrial Premature Complexes:." Pacing and Clinical Electrophysiology 27.2 (2004).

Sunbul, M., O. Erdogan, and B. Mutlu. "Torsade de pointes." Herz 38.4 (2013): 423-426.

Skouibine, Kirill, Natalia Trayanova, and Peter Moore. "Success and Failure of the Defibrillation Shock:." Journal of Cardiovascular Electrophysiology 11.7 (2000).

Jambukia, Shweta H., Vipul K. Dabhi, and Harshadkumar B. Prajapati. "ECG beat classification using machine learning techniques." International Journal of Biomedical Engineering and Technology 26.1 (2018): 32-53.

Roshan, John, Andrew C.T. Ha, Krishnakumar Nair, and Vijay S. Chauhan. "Paroxysmal Tachycardia with Pauses to Ponder." Journal of Cardiovascular Electrophysiology 24.1 (2013).

Monfredi, Oliver, Halina Dobrzynski, Tapas Mondal, Mark R. Boyett, and Gwilym M. Morris. "The Anatomy and Physiology of the Sinoatrial Node—A Contemporary Review." Pacing and Clinical Electrophysiology 33.11 (2010).

Plumb, Vance. "Atrial Flutter." Cardiac Electrophysiology Review 3.2 (2004): 113-114.

Un, Haluk, Mehmet Dogan, Omer Uz, Zafer Isilak, and Mehmet Uzun. "Novel vagal maneuver technique for termination of supraventricular tachycardias." The American Journal of Emergency Medicine 34.1 (2016): 118.e5-118.e7.

"Premature Ventricular Complex Morphology." Circulation 81.4 (1990): 1245-1251.

Alraies, M. Chadi, Naseem Eisa, Abdul Hamid Alraiyes, and Khaldoon Shaheen. "The Long and Short of It: Ashman's Phenomenon." The American Journal of Medicine 126.11 (2013): 962-963.

Grimm, Wolfram. "Accelerated Idioventricular Rhythm." Cardiac Electrophysiology Review 5.3 (2004): 328-331.

Talwar, K., and N. Naik. "Etiology and Management of Sustained Ventricular Tachycardia." American Journal of Cardiovascular Drugs 1.3 (2012): 179-192.

Brady, William J, and Jeff Skiles. "Wide QRS complex tachycardia: ECG differential diagnosis." The American Journal of Emergency Medicine 17.4 (1999): 376-381.

Nichol, Graham, Michael R. Sayre, Federico Guerra, and Jeanne Poole. "Defibrillation for Ventricular Fibrillation." Journal of the American College of Cardiology 70.12 (2017): A1-A30.

Futrell, Amelia G., "Decreased Cardiac Output." Dimensions of Critical Care Nursing 9.4 (1990): 202-208.

Chapter 8

El-Segaier, Milad, and Gudrun Björkhem. "Complete atrio-ventricular septal defect and Wolf-Parkinson-White syndrome." The Libyan Journal of Medicine 1.2 (2006): 185-189.

Yanai, Seika, Yasuhiro Ishikawa, Shigeto Fuse, and Hiroyuki Tsutsumi. "Inverse Independent Component Analysis Facilitates Clarification of the Accessory Conductive Pathway of Wolf–Parkinson–White Syndrome Electrocardiogram." Pediatric Cardiology 30.1 (2008): 59-69.

Malagoli, Alessandro, Luca Rossi, Caterina Mastrojanni, and Giovanni Quinto Villani. "A perfect storm: Wolf Parkinson White syndrome, Ebstein's anomaly, biventricular non-compaction, and bicuspid aortic valve." European Heart Journal – Cardiovascular Imaging 15.7 (2014): 827-827.

CastellanoS, Agustin, Liaqat Zaman, Federigo Moleiro, Juan M. Aranda, and Robert J. Myerburg. "The Lown-Ganong-Levine Syndrome." Pacing and Clinical Electrophysiology 5.5 (1982).

Bhargava, Kartikeya, Sameer Shrivastava, Balbir Singh, and Hein J. Wellens. "AV block. Which type and where?." Journal of Electrocardiology 40.4 (2007): 358-359.

Ho, Reginald T., Matthew Stopper, and Anish R. Koka. "Alternating Bundle Branch Block." Pacing and Clinical Electrophysiology 35.2 (2012).

Siliste, Calin, Maria-Claudia-Berenice Suran, Andrei-Dumitru Margulescu, and Dragos Vinereanu. "Right Ventricular Electrical and Mechanical Synchronization by Properly Timed Septal Pacing in a Patient with Right Bundle Branch Block and First Degree AV Block—A Case Report." Annals of Noninvasive Electrocardiology 20.2 (2015): 193-197.

Littmann, Laszlo, and J. Warren Holshouser. "Not so Fast: Acceleration-dependent or Mobitz Type II Second-degree AV Block." The American Journal of Medicine 125.10 (2012): 967-970.

Huang, Weiting, Paul Chun Yih Lim, and Chi-Keong Ching. "Wenckebach pattern in right bundle branch block – benign or not?." Journal of Electrocardiology 50.2 (2017): 223-226.

Kawai, Sachio, Lontai Fu, Kousuke Aziki, Ryozo Okada, and Kazuzo Katoh. "A Degenerative

Lesion of the Approach to the Atrioventricular Node Producing Second-Degree and Third-Degree Atrioventricular Block." Pacing and Clinical Electrophysiology 15.12 (1992).

Josephson, Mark E., and Hein J.J. Wellens. "The ECG in left bundle branch block and heart failure." Heart Rhythm 12.1 (2015): 250-251.

Galeotti, Loriano, Peter M. van Dam, Zak Loring, Dulciana Chan, and David G. Strauss. "Evaluating strict and conventional left bundle branch block criteria using electrocardiographic simulations." Europace 15.12 (2013): 1816-1821.

Rickard, John, Dharam J. Kumbhani, Eiran Z. Gorodeski, Bryan Baranowski, Oussama Wazni, David O. martin, Richard Grimm, and Bruce L. Wilkoff. "Cardiac Resynchronization Therapy in Non-Left Bundle Branch Block Morphologies." Pacing and Clinical Electrophysiology 33.5 (2010).

Madias, John E. "Mechanism of transient resolution of chronic complete right bundle branch block following an acute anterior myocardial infarction." Journal of Electrocardiology 48.5 (2015).

Aizawa, Yoshiyasu, Seiji Takatsuki, Takehiro Kimura, Nobuhiro Nishiyama, Kotaro Fukumoto, Yoko Tanimoto, Kojiro Tanimoto, Shunichiro Miyoshi, Makoto Suzuki, Yasuhiro Yokoyama, Masaomi Chinushi, Ichiro Watanabe, Satoshi Ogawa, Yoshifusa Aizawa, Charles Antzelevitch, and Keiichi Fukuda. "Ventricular fibrillation associated with complete right bundle branch block." Heart Rhythm 10.7 (2013): 1028-1035.

Lim, Ven Gee, Kay Por Yip, Zhan Yun Lim, Simon Sporton, and Simon Kennon. "The 'Normal' Heart: Fascicular Ventricular Tachycardia." The American Journal of Medicine 129.6 (2016): 580-582.

Shah, Bimal R., Christine Lin, Charles Maynard, Bradley Bart, Ronald H. Selvester, Linda K. Shaw, Christopher O'Connor, and Galen S. Wagner. "Specificity of electrocardiographic myocardial infarction screening criteria in patients with nonischemic cardiomyopathies." American Heart Journal 136.2 (1998): 314-319.

Bayés de Luna, Antonio, Andrés Pérez Riera, Adrian Baranchuk, Pablo Chiale, Pedro Iturralde, Carlos Pastore, Raimundo Barbosa, Diego Goldwasser, Paolo Alboni, and Marcelo Elizari. "Electrocardiographic manifestation of the middle fibers/septal fascicle block: a consensus report." Journal of Electrocardiology 45.5 (2012): 454-460.

Olson, Charles W., David Lange, Jack-Kang Chan, Kim E. Olson, Alfred Albano, Galen S. Wagner, and Ronald H.S. Selvester. "3D Heart: A new visual training method for Electrocardiographic Analysis." Journal of Electrocardiology 40.5 (2007): 457.e1-457.e7.

Pérez-Riera, Andres Ricardo, and Adrian Baranchuk. "Unusual Conduction Disorder: Left Posterior Fascicular Block + Left Septal Fascicular Block." Annals of Noninvasive Electrocardiology 20.2 (2015): 187-188.

Cappato, Riccardo. "The case of chronic bifascicular block: still a worrying ECG finding?." Europace 11.9 (2009): 1140-1141.

Lichstein, Edgar, Prem K. Gupta, and Kul D. Chadda. "Indications for Pacing in Patients with Chronic Bifascicular Block." Pacing and Clinical Electrophysiology 1.4 (1978).

Seewoodhary, J., and L. Griffin. "Trifascicular block and a raised Troponin T in acute cholecystitis." QJM: An International Journal of Medicine 103.2 (2010): 121-123.

Ibarrola, Martín, Pablo Ambrosio Chiale, Andrés Ricardo Pérez-Riera, and Adrian Baranchuk. "Phase 4 left septal fascicular block." Heart Rhythm 11.9 (2014): 1655-1657.

Kumar, Ashish, Rama Komaragiri, and Manjeet Kumar. "From Pacemaker to Wearable: Techniques for ECG Detection Systems." Journal of Medical Systems 42.2 (2018): 1-17.

Tran, Viet, Tracy Holt, and Yochai Birnbaum. "What is causing the finding: the pacemaker, patient or the ECG machine?." Journal of Electrocardiology 47.5 (2014): 752-754.

Kong, Chi-Woon, Ta-Chuan Tuan, Wei-Hsian Yin, Wen-Chung Yu, Shih-Ann Chen, Yenn-Jiang Lin, Chun-Yao Huang, and Sheng-Liang Chung. "Development of Atrial Fibrillation in Patients with Atrioventricular Block After Atrioventricular Synchronized Pacing." Pacing and Clinical Electrophysiology 27.3 (2004).

Hong, Paul S.G., Guy Amit, Jeff S. Healey, and Syamkumar Divakara Menon. "Consistent Inconsistency? Is There Pacemaker Malfunction?." Journal of Cardiovascular Electrophysiology 27.1 (2016): 131-133.

Littmann, Laszlo, and Robert M. Farrell. "Potential misinterpretations related to artificial pacemaker signals generated by electrocardiographs." Journal of Electrocardiology 48.4 (2015): 717-720.

Pérez, Óscar Cano, María José Sancho-Tello de Carranza, Joaquín Osca Asensi, and José A. Olagüe de Ros. "Pacemaker malfunction or non-physiological ventricular pacing?." Europace 10.2 (2008): 161-163.

Matusik, Paweł T., Andrzej Ząbek, Patrycja S. Matusik, Barbara Małecka, and Jacek Lelakowski. "Atrioventricular synchrony in the background of ventricular noise and undersensing." Annals of Noninvasive Electrocardiology 22.4 (2017): n/a-n/a.

Lesh, Michael D., Jonathan J. Langberg, Jerry C. Griffin, Melvin M. Scheinman, and Charles L. Witherell. "Pacemaker Generator Pseudomalfunction: An Artifact of Holter Monitoring." Pacing and Clinical Electrophysiology 14.5 (1991).

Chapter 9

Tsioufis, Costas, George Lazaros, Dimitrios Vassilopoulos, Panagiotis Vasileiou, and Christodoulos Stefanadis. "ECG Changes Mimicking Myocardial Infarction." The American Journal of Medicine 123.11 (2010): 996-998.

Erdogan, Okan, Bahar Dalkilic, and Alper Kepez. "Horizontal ECG in acute anterolateral myocardial infarction." Wiener klinische Wochenschrift 128.14 (2016): 524-527.

Kumar, Arun, Subrata Kar, and William P. Fay. "Thrombosis, physical activity, and acute coronary syndromes." Journal of Applied Physiology 111.2 (2011)599.

Jackson, Shaun P. "Arterial thrombosis—insidious, unpredictable and deadly." Nature Medicine 17.11 (2011): 1423-1436.

"Risk Factors For Coronary Disease." Journal of American Geriatrics Society 16.5 (1968): 628-629.

Zengin, Elvin, Christoph Bickel, Renate B. Schnabel, Tanja Zeller, Karl-J. Lackner, Hans-J. Rupprecht, Stefan Blankenberg, Dirk Westermann, and Dirk Westermann. "Risk Factors of Coronary Artery Disease in Secondary Prevention—Results from the Athero Gene —Study." PLoS ONE 10.7 (2015).

Merz, MDC.Noel Bairey, Alan MDRozanski, and James S. MDForrester. "The Secondary Prevention of Coronary Artery Disease." The American Journal of Medicine 102.6 (1997): 572-581.

Childers, Rory. "R wave amplitude in ischemia, injury, and infarction." Journal of Electrocardiology 29 (1996): 171-178.

Hoit, Brian D. "Pathophysiology of the Pericardium." Progress in Cardiovascular Diseases 59.4 (2017): 341-348.

Irina, Pintilie, Scridon Alina, and Şerban Răzvan Constantin. "To Be or Not to Be ... Acute Coronary Syndrome." Acta Medica Marisiensis 62.3 (2016).

Giugliano, Robert P., and Eugene Braunwald. "The Year in Acute Coronary Syndrome." Journal of the American College of Cardiology 63.3 (2014): 201-214.

Carreiro-Lewandowski, Eileen. "Update on Cardiac Biomarkers." Laboratory Medicine 37.10 (2006): 597-605.

Birnbaum, Yochai, James Michael Wilson, Miquel Fiol, Antonio Bayés Luna, Markku Eskola, and Kjell Nikus. "ECG Diagnosis and Classification of Acute Coronary Syndromes." Annals of Noninvasive Electrocardiology 19.1 (2014): 4-14.

Gonzalez, Jorge, and George Beller. "Choosing exercise or pharmacologic stress imaging, or exercise ECG testing alone: How to decide." Journal of Nuclear Cardiology 24.2 (2016): 555-557.

Kaluzay, Jozef, Katleen Vandenberghe, Damien Fontaine, Lieven Herbots, Anné Wim, Frans Van de Werf, and Hein Heidbüchel. "ST-deviation reconstruction in missing leads on the 12-lead ECG: applicability in studies on ST-segment resolution during thrombolysis." Journal of Electrocardiology 36.3 (2003): 187-193.

Guo, Xiao Hua, Yee Guan, Li Jia Chen, Jian Huang, and A. John Camm. "Correlation of coronary angiography with "tombstoning" electrocardiographic pattern in patients after acute myocardial infarction." Clinical Cardiology 23.5 (2000): 347-352.

Nable, Jose Victor, and William Brady. "The evolution of electrocardiographic changes in ST-segment elevation myocardial infarction." The American Journal of Emergency Medicine 27.6 (2009): 734-746.

Michael, Mark A., Hicham El Masry, Bilal R. Khan, and Mithilesh K. Das. "Electrocardiographic Signs of Remote Myocardial Infarction." Progress in Cardiovascular Diseases 50.3 (2007): 198-208.

Karnath, Bernard M, John C Champion, and Masood Ahmad. "Electrocardiographic manifestions of proximal left anterior descending artery occlusion." Journal of Electrocardiology 36.2 (2003): 173-177.

Raitt, Merritt H., Paul F. Litwin, Jenny S. Martin, and W. Douglas Weaver. "ECG findings in acute myocardial infarction." Journal of Electrocardiology 28.1 (1995): 13-16.

Wellens, Hein J. "An inferior myocardial infarction with conduction abnormalities." Heart Rhythm 15.1 (2018): 151-152.

Huang, Xin, Sachin K. Ramdhany, Yong Zhang, Zuyi Yuan, Gary S. Mintz, and Ning Guo. "New ST-segment algorithms to determine culprit artery location in acute inferior myocardial infarction." The American Journal of Emergency Medicine 34.9 (2016): 1772-1778.

Goldberg, Alexander, Danielle A. Southern, P. Diane Galbraith, Mouhieddin Traboulsi, Merril L. Knudtson, and William A. Ghali. "Coronary dominance and prognosis of patients with acute coronary syndrome." American Heart Journal 154.6 (2007): 1116-1122.

Bengal, Tuvia, Itzhak Herz, Alejandro Solodky, Yochai Birnbaum, Samuel Sclarovsky, and Alex Sagie. "Acute anterior wall myocardial infarction entailing st-segment elevation in lead v 1 : Electrocardiographic and angiographic correlations." Clinical Cardiology 21.6 (1998): 399-404.

Littmann, Laszlo. "The Dressler - de Winter sign of acute proximal LAD occlusion." Journal of Electrocardiology 51.1 (2018): 138-139.

Rhinehardt, Joseph, William J. Brady, Andrew D. Perron, and Amal Mattu. "Electrocardiographic manifestations of Wellens' syndrome." The American Journal of Emergency Medicine 20.7 (2002): 638-643.

Wiiala, Jonathan, Erik Hedström, Morten Kraen, Martin Magnusson, Håkan Arheden, and Henrik Engblom. "Diagnostic performance of the Selvester QRS scoring system in relation to clinical ECG assessment of patients with lateral myocardial infarction using cardiac magnetic resonance as reference standard." Journal of Electrocardiology 48.5 (2015): 750-757.

Brady, William J, Brian Erling, Marc Pollack, and Theodore C Chan. "Electrocardiographic manifestations: Acute posterior wall myocardial infarction." Journal of Emergency Medicine 20.4 (2001): 391-401.

Lim, Soo-Teik, and James Goldstein. "Right ventricular infarction." Current Treatment Options in Cardiovascular Medicine 3.2 (2001): 95-101.

Eskola, Markku J., Petteri Kosonen, Samuel Sclarovsky, Saila Vikman, and Kjell C. Nikus. "The ECG Pattern of Isolated Right Ventricular Infarction during Percutaneous Coronary Intervention." Annals of Noninvasive Electrocardiology 12.1 (2007).

Madias, John E. "Serial ECG recordings via marked chest wall landmarks: An essential requirement for the diagnosis of myocardial infarction in the presence of left bundle branch block." Journal of Electrocardiology 35.4 (2002): 299-302.

Smith SW, Dodd KW, Henry TD, Dvorak DM, and Pearce LA. "Diagnosis of ST-elevation myocardial infarction in the presence of left bundle branch block with the ST-elevation to S-wave ratio in a modified Sgarbossa rule. Annals of Emergency Medicine 60.6 (2012): 766-776.

Sefa, Nana, and Kelly N. Sawyer. "Smith-Modified Sgarbossa Criteria and Paced Rhythms: A Case Report." Journal of Emergency Medicine 51.5 (2016): 584-588.

Briller, Stanley A. "Important Uses of Electrocardiography." AJN, American Journal of Nursing 55.11 (1955).

Hetland, Mathias, Kristina H. Haugaa, Sebastian I. Sarvari, Gunnar Erikssen, Erik Kongsgaard, and Thor Edvardsen. "A Novel ECG-Index for Prediction of Ventricular Arrhythmias in Patients after Myocardial Infarction." Annals of Noninvasive Electrocardiology 19.4 (2014): 330-337.

Castle, Nick. "Reperfusion therapy." Emergency Nurse 13.9 (2006): 25-35.

Boersma, Eric, Ewout Steyerberg, Maureen Vlugt, and Maarten Simoons. "Reperfusion Therapy for Acute Myocardial Infarction." Drugs 56.1 (2012): 31-48.

Rheuban, Karen. "Pericarditis." Current Treatment Options in Cardiovascular Medicine 7.5 (2005): 419-427.

Chhabra, Lovely, and B. M. Pamapana Gowd. "Hypothermia Can Masquerade as Pericarditis: Yet Another Possibility to be Considered in the Differential Diagnosis." Journal of Emergency Medicine 50.3 (2016): e171-e172.

Drifmeyer, Erin, and Kenneth Batts. "The Brugada syndrome." Current Sports Medicine Reports 4.2 (2014): 83-87.

Kono, Tatsuji, and Hani Sabbah. "Takotsubo cardiomyopathy." Heart Failure Reviews 19.5 (2013): 585-593.

Ghadri, J.R., F. Ruschitzka, T.F. Lscher, and C. Templin. "Prinzmetal angina." QJM: An International Journal of Medicine 107.5 (2014): 375-377.

Macfarlane, Peter W., Charles Antzelevitch, Michel Haissaguerre, Heikki V. Huikuri, Mark Potse, Raphael Rosso, Frederic Sacher, Jani T. Tikkanen, Hein Wellens, and Gan-Xin Yan. "The Early Repolarization Pattern." Journal of the American College of Cardiology 66.4 (2015): 470-477.

Chapter 10

Freeman, Kalev, James A. Feldman, Patricia Mitchell, Jacqueline Donovan, K. Sophia Dyer, Laura Eliseo, Laura Forsberg White, and Elizabeth S. Temin. "Effects of Presentation and Electrocardiogram on Time to Treatment of Hyperkalemia." Academic Emergency Medicine 15.3 (2008).

Hlaing, Thinn, Tara DiMino, Peter R. Kowey, and Gan-Xin Yan. "ECG Repolarization Waves: Their Genesis and Clinical Implications." Annals of Noninvasive Electrocardiology 10.2 (2005).

Chorin, Ehud, Raphael Rosso, and Sami Viskin. "Electrocardiographic Manifestations of Calcium Abnormalities." Annals of Noninvasive Electrocardiology 21.1 (2016): 7-9.

Azie, Nkechi E., Gregory Adams, Borje Darpo, Steven F. Francom, Emery C. Polasek, Joy M. Wisser, and Joseph C. Fleishaker. "Comparing Methods of Measurement for Detecting Drug-Induced Changes in the QT Interval: Implications for Thoroughly Conducted ECG Studies." Annals of Noninvasive Electrocardiology 9.2 (2004).

Nada, Adel, Gary A. Gintant, Robert Kleiman, David E. Gutstein, Christer Gottfridsson, Eric L. Michelson, Colette Strnadova, Matthew Killeen, Mary Jane Geiger, Mónica L. Fiszman, Luana Pesco Koplowitz, Glenn F. Carlson, Ignacio Rodriguez, and Philip T. Sager. "The evaluation and management of drug effects on cardiac conduction (PR and QRS Intervals) in clinical development." American Heart Journal 165.4 (2013): 489-500.

Morita, Hiroshi, Shiho Takenaka Morita, Satoshi Nagase, Kimikazu Banba, Nobuhiro Nishii, Yoshinori Tani, Atsuyuki Watanabe, Kazufumi Nakamura, Kengo Fukushima Kusano, Tetsuro Emori, Hiromi Matsubara, Kazumasa Hina, Toshimasa Kita, and Tohru Ohe. "Ventricular arrhythmia induced by sodium channel blocker in patients with Brugada syndrome." Journal of the American College of Cardiology 42.9 (2003): 1624-1631.

Khan, Ijaz A., and Chandra K. Nair. "Brugada and Long QT-3 Syndromes: Two Phenotypes of the Sodium Channel Disease." Annals of Noninvasive Electrocardiology 9.3 (2004).

Scholz, H. "Classification and mechanism of action of antiarrhythmic drugs *." Fundamental & Clinical Pharmacology 8.5 (1994).

Nicole Schmitt, Morten GrunnetSøren-Peter Olesen. "Cardiac Potassium Channel Subtypes: New Roles in Repolarization and Arrhythmia." Physiological Reviews 94.2 (2014)609.

Reiter, Michael J., and James A. Reiffel. "Importance of beta blockade in the therapy of serious ventricular arrhythmias." The American Journal of Cardiology 82.4 (1998): 9I-19I.

Herweg, Bengt, Arzu Ilercil, Ray Cutro, Robert Dewhurst, Sendhil Krishnan, Mark Weston, and S. Serge Barold. "Cardiac Resynchronization Therapy in Patients With End-Stage Inotrope-Dependent Class IV Heart Failure." The American Journal of Cardiology 100.1 (2007): 90-93.

Ahmed, Ali, MD, MPH, Mihai Gheorghiade, MD, William H. Wehrmacher, MD and Michel White, and MD. "The Role of Digoxin in Heart Failure." The Medical Roundtable Cardiovascular Edition 1.3 (2010): 176-181.

Steg, Philippe. "Stable Angina." American Journal of Cardiovascular Drugs 3.1 (2012): 1-10.

Boniface, Keith S., and James A. Feldman. "Thrombolytic therapy and cocaine-associated acute myocardial infarction." The American Journal of Emergency Medicine 18.5 (2000): 612-615.

Ullman, Edward, William J. Brady, Andrew D. Perron, Theodore Chan, and Amal Mattu. "Electrocardiographic manifestations of pulmonary embolism." The American Journal of Emergency Medicine 19.6 (2001): 514-519.

Zhang, Jinghua, Guizhi Liu, Suifeng Wang, Weiguo Du, Peisheng Lv, Hua Guo, Qian Sun, Yining Liu, and Xinxin Qi. "The electrocardiographic characteristics of an acute embolism in the pulmonary trunk and the main pulmonary arteries." The American Journal of Emergency Medicine 34.2 (2016): 212-217.

Willis Hurst, J., Rajagopal Baliepally, and David H. Spodick Fccp. "Electrocardiographic screening for emphysema: The frontal plane p axis." Clinical Cardiology 22.3 (1999): 226-228.

Thomas, Anish J., Sirin Apiyasawat, and David H. Spodick. "Electrocardiographic Detection of Emphysema." The American Journal of Cardiology 107.7 (2011): 1090-1092.

Fox, N., and N. Sadick. "Electrocardiographic changes in hypothermia." Internal Medicine Journal 38.7 (2008).

Federman, Nicholas J., Alexis Mechulan, George J. Klein, and Andrew D. Krahn. "Ventricular Fibrillation Induced by Spontaneous Hypothermia in a Patient with Early Repolarization Syndrome." Journal of Cardiovascular Electrophysiology 24.5 (2013): 586-588.

Pillarisetti, Jayasree, and Kamal Gupta. "Giant Inverted T waves in the emergency department: case report and review of differential diagnoses." Journal of Electrocardiology 43.1 (2010): 40-42.

Pauschinger, M., M. Noutsias, D. Lassner, H.-P. Schultheiss, and U. Kuehl. "Inflammation, ECG changes and pericardial effusion." Zeitschrift für Kardiologie 95.11 (2006): 569-583.

Baggish, Aaron L. "A decade of athlete ECG criteria: Where we've come and where we're going." Journal of Electrocardiology 48.3 (2015): 324-328.

Campbell, Matthew J., Xuefu Zhou, Chia Han, Hedayat Abrishami, Gregory Webster, Christina Y. Miyake, Christopher T. Sower, Jeffrey B. Anderson, Timothy K. Knilans, and Richard J. Czosek. "Pilot study analyzing automated ECG screening of hypertrophic cardiomyopathy." Heart Rhythm 14.6 (2017): A1-A20.

Behr, Elijah, and William McKenna. "Hypertrophic Cardiomyopathy." Current Treatment Options in Cardiovascular Medicine 4.6 (2002): 443-453.

Perazzolo Marra, M., S. Rizzo, B. Bauce, M. De Lazzari, K. Pilichou, D. Corrado, G. Thiene, S. Iliceto, and C. Basso. "Arrhythmogenic right ventricular cardiomyopathy." Herz 40.4 (2015): 600-606.

Steriotis, Alexandros Klavdios, Barbara Bauce, Luciano Daliento, Ilaria Rigato, Elisa Mazzotti, Antonio Franco Folino, Martina Perazzolo Marra, Luca Brugnaro, and Andrea Nava. "Electrocardiographic Pattern in Arrhythmogenic Right Ventricular Cardiomyopathy." The American Journal of Cardiology 103.9 (2009): 1302-1308.

Obeyesekere, Manoj N., Simon Modi, and George J. Klein. "Concealed Conduction." Journal of Cardiovascular Electrophysiology 22.12 (2011).

Kinoshita, Shinji, Takao Mitsuoka, Takakazu Katoh, and Yohtaro Oyama. "Concealed conduction in the reentrant pathway as a mechanism of stable ventricular quadrigeminy." Journal of Electrocardiology 33.1 (2000): 93-97.

Chapter 11

Pelliccia, Antonio, Martin S. Maron, and Barry J. Maron. "Assessment of Left Ventricular Hypertrophy in a Trained Athlete: Differential Diagnosis of Physiologic Athlete's Heart From Pathologic Hypertrophy." Progress in Cardiovascular Diseases 54.5 (2012): 387-396.

Malagoli, Alessandro, Luca Rossi, Caterina Mastrojanni, and Giovanni Quinto Villani. "A perfect storm: Wolf Parkinson White syndrome, Ebstein's anomaly, biventricular non-compaction, and bicuspid aortic valve." European Heart Journal – Cardiovascular Imaging 15.7 (2014): 827-827.

Szabo, Tibor S., George J. Klein, Gerard M. Guiraudon, Raymond Yee, and Arjun D. Sharma. "Localization of Accessory Pathways in the Wolff-Parkinson-White Syndrome." Pacing and Clinical Electrophysiology 12.10 (1989).

Ehara, Shoichi, Takao Hasegawa, Kenji Matsumoto, Kenichiro Otsuka, Takanori Yamazaki, Tomokazu Iguchi, Yasukatsu Izumi, Kenei Shimada, and Minoru Yoshiyama. "The strain pattern, and not Sokolow–Lyon electrocardiographic voltage criteria, is independently associated with anatomic left ventricular hypertrophy." Heart and Vessels 29.5 (2013): 638-644.

Brugada, Josep. "Relevance of Atrial Fibrillation Classification in Clinical Practice." Journal of Cardiovascular Electrophysiology 13.S1 (2002): S27-S30.

Ng, Geelyn J.L., Amy M.L. Quek, Christine Cheung, Thiruma V. Arumugam, and Raymond C.S. Seet. "Stroke biomarkers in clinical practice: A critical appraisal." Neurochemistry International 107 (2017): 11-22.

Cairns, John A. "The search for the ideal atrial fibrillation stroke risk prediction schema: is ATRIA a contender?." European Heart Journal 37.42 (2016): 3211-3212.

Bloom, Heather L. "Concise review of atrial fibrillation: Treatment update considerations in light of AFFIRM and RACE." Clinical Cardiology 27.9 (2004): 495-500.

Rijnbeek, Peter R., Gerard van Herpen, Michiel L. Bots, Sumche Man, Niek Verweij, Albert Hofman, Hans Hillege, Matthijs E. Numans, Cees A. Swenne, Jacqueline C.M. Witteman, and Jan A. Kors. "Normal values of the electrocardiogram for ages 16–90 years." Journal of Electrocardiology 47.6 (2014): 914-921.

Shukla, Ashish, and Anne B Curtis. "Avoiding permanent atrial fibrillation: treatment approaches to prevent disease progression." Vascular Health and Risk Management 10 (2014): 1-12.

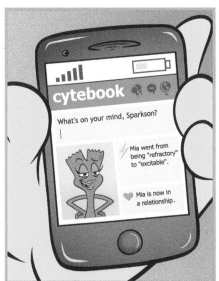
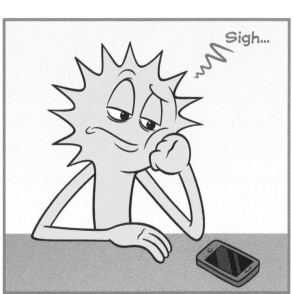
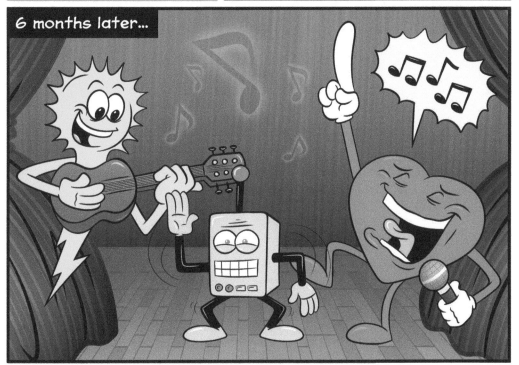
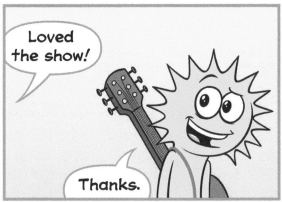
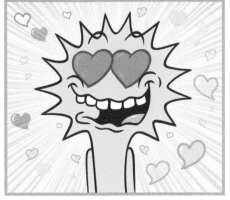

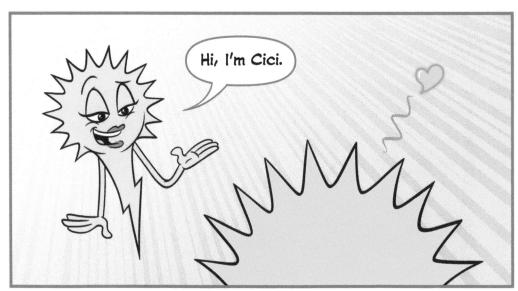

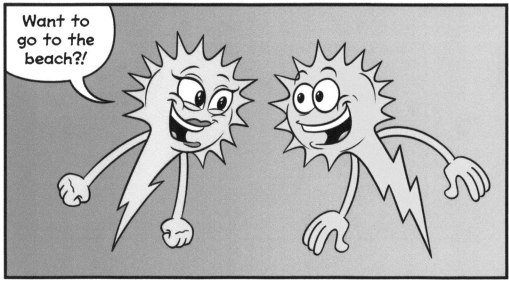

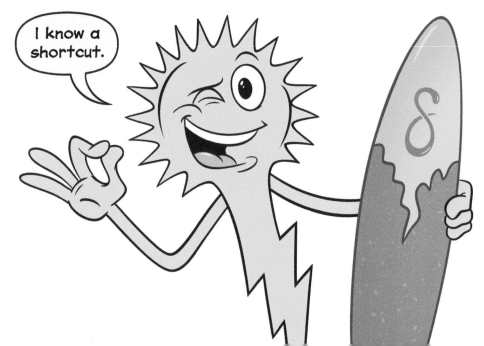

INDEX

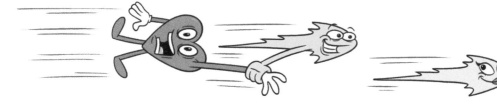

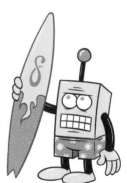

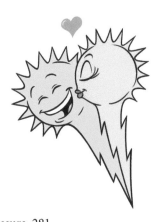

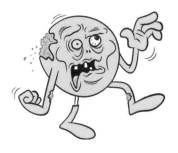

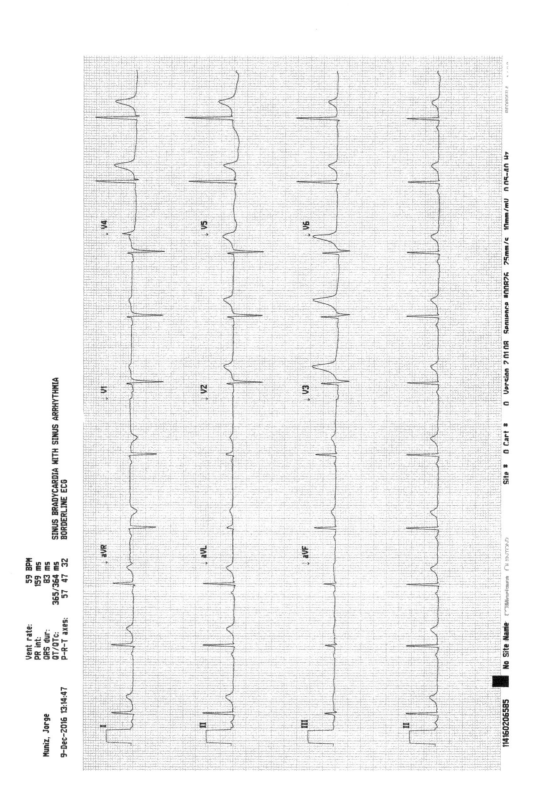

Muniz, Jorge

9-Dec-2016 13:14:47

Vent rate: 59 BPM
PR int: 159 ms
QRS dur: 83 ms
QT/QTc: 365/364 ms
P-R-T axes: 57 47 32

SINUS BRADYCARDIA WITH SINUS ARRHYTHMIA
BORDERLINE ECG

No Site Name

Site # 0 Cart # 0 Version 2.01.08 Sequence #00826 25mm/s 10mm/mV 0.05-40 Hz

114160206585

CPSIA information can be obtained
at www.ICGtesting.com
Printed in the USA
LVHW010712220321
682049LV00007B/27

9 780996 651370